Depression:
Social and Economic Timebomb

Depression:
Social and Economic
Timebomb

Strategies for quality care

Proceedings of an international meeting

Organised by the World Health Organization in collaboration with the
International Federation of Health Funds, Harvard Medical School and the
Sir Robert Mond Memorial Trust

Chaired by Arthur Kleinman MD

Edited by

ANN DAWSON MD and ANDRE TYLEE MD

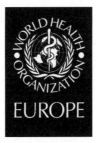

Published on behalf of the World Health Organization
Regional office for Europe by BMJ Books

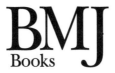

First published in 2001
by the BMJ Publishing Group, BMA House, Tavistock Square,
London WC1H 9JR

British Library Cataloguing in Publication Data

A catalogue record for this book is available from the British Library

ISBN 0-7279-1573-8

Cover design by Goodall James, Dorset
Typeset by FiSH Books, London
Printed and bound by J W Arrowsmith Ltd, Bristol

Contents

DEPRESSION AND GENERAL PRACTICE

DEPRESSION AND THE WORKPLACE

*Note: these sections were not part of the proceedings

ECONOMIC AND SOCIETAL CONSEQUENCES

THE DEBATE

CLOSING REMARKS OF THE MEETING   177

Contributors

David Ames MD Professor of Psychiatry of Old Age, Royal Park Hospital, Victoria, Australia

Jo Erik Asvall MD WHO Regional Director for Europe, World Health Organization Regional Office for Europe, Copenhagen, Denmark

Per Bech MD Director, WHO Collaborating Centre for Mental Health, Psychiatric Research Unit, Frederiksborg General Hospital, Hillerød, Denmark

Ernst R Berndt PhD Professor of Applied Economics, AP Sloan School of Management, Massachusetts Institute of Technology, USA; Director, Program on Technological Progress and Productivity Measurement, National Bureau of Economic Research, Cambridge, Massachusetts, USA

Somnath Chatterji MD Scientist, Classification, Assessment, Surveys and Terminology Team, World Health Organization, Geneva, Switzerland

Daniel Chisholm MSc Economist, Classification, Assessment, Surveys and Terminology Team, AS Group, World Health Organization, Geneva, Switzerland

Alex Cohen PhD Anthropologist and Instructor in Social Medicine, Department of Social Medicine, Harvard Medical School, Boston, USA

John Cox MD President, Royal College of Psychiatrists, Professor of Psychiatry, School of Postgraduate Medicine, Keele University, Stoke on Trent, United Kingdom

Ann Dawson MD Director, World Health Organization Office for Quality in Non-Communicable Diseases & Conditions, London, United Kingdom

John Donoghue BSc MRPharmS Honorary Lecturer School of Pharmacy and Chemistry, Liverpool John Moores University, Liverpool, United Kingdom

John Geddes MD Senior Clinical Research Fellow, Honorary Consultant Psychiatrist and Director, Centre for Evidence Based Mental Health, University Department of Psychiatry, Warneford Hospital, Oxford, United Kingdom

David Healy MD Consultant Psychiatrist, Director, North Wales Department of Psychological Medicine, Hergest Unit, Bangor, United Kingdom

Kevin Holland-Elliott MD Director and Consultant, Department of Occupational Health Safety, Kings College Hospital, London, United Kingdom

Richard Hornsby Chief Executive, The Sir Robert Mond Memorial Trust, London, United Kingdom

Allan House MD Professor of Psychiatry, University of Leeds, Leeds, United Kingdom

Peter Juhn PhD Executive Director, Care Management Institute, Kaiser Foundation Health Plan Inc, Oakland, USA

Yves Lecrubier MD Director, INSERM, Hôpital le Salpêtrière, Paris, France

Sir Denis Pereira Gray OBE MD President Royal College of Psychiatrists, Professor of General Practice, University of Exeter, Exeter, United Kingdom and President, Royal College of General Practitioners **Steven Reid** MD Clinical Research Fellow, Academic Department of Psychological Medicine, Guys, Kings and St Thomas' School of Medicine, Institute of Psychiatry, London, United Kingdom

Wolfgang Rutz MD Regional Adviser in Mental Health, WHO Regional Office for Europe, World Health Organization, Copenhagen, Denmark

Tom Sackville Chief Executive, International Federation of Health Funds, London, United Kingdom

David Alexander Sclar PhD Boeing Distinguished Professor of Health & Policy Administration, Boehringer Ingelheim Scholar in Pharmaceutical Economics, Director, Pharmacoeconomics and Pharmacoepidemiology Research Unit, College of Pharmacy, Washington State University, Pullman, Washington, USA

Edward Shorter PhD Professor of the History of Medicine, History of Medicine Programme, University of Toronto, Toronto, Ontario, Canada

Kirsten Staehr Johansen MD WHO Consultant, Country Health Programme, World Health Organization Regional Office for Europe, Copenhagen, Denmark

Andre Tylee MD Professor of Primary Care Mental Health at the Institute of Psychiatry, Kings College, London, United Kingdom

T Bedirhan Üstün MD Group Leader, Classification, Assessment, Surveys and Terminology Team, World Health Organization, Geneva, Switzerland

Simon Wessely MD Professor of Epidemiological and Liaison Psychiatry, Academic Department of Psychological Medicine, Guys, Kings and St Thomas' School of Medicine, Institute of Psychiatry, London, United Kingdom

Overall Chairman: Arthur Kleinman MD

Arthur Kleinman MD, Maude and Lillian Presley Professor of Medical Anthropology, Professor of Psychiatry, and Chairman, Department of Social Medicine, Harvard Medical School, and Professor of Social Anthropology, Department of Anthropology, Faculty of Arts and Sciences, Harvard University, has conducted cross-cultural research since 1968 on illness experience and health care in Chinese society and North America.

The author of more than 150 articles; author of 5 books; and editor or co-editor of 15 volumes; Kleinman has directed the World Mental Health Report, supported by Carnegie Corporation, MacArthur and Rockefeller Foundations and the Milbank Fund. He was a member of the Steering Committee of the American Psychiatric Association-National Institute of Mental Health Taskforce on Culture and Psychiatric Diagnosis, and Co-Chair, Committee on Culture, Health and Human Development, Social Science Research Council.

1O DOWNING STREET
LONDON SW1A 2AA

THE PRIME MINISTER

Promoting good mental health and preventing mental ill health benefits all of us. Depression is a particular concern, which costs lives, and affects the quality of life. We can achieve the goals we set in *Saving Lives*, and we can realise our ambitions for modernising health and social care services, but only if we tackle the underlying social economic and environmental conditions as well as the specific causes.

I congratulate you on your initiative in developing the Ludwig Mond Medal award to recognise excellence in industry in this important area, and wish you all the best for a very successful conference.

Tony Blair

October 1999

Editorial note:

The Ludwig Mond Medal is an international award that recognises excellence and achievement by a leader of industry in relation to wellbeing in the work place and is presented annually by the Society of Chemical Industry.

Acknowledgement

Grateful acknowledgement is hereby made to all those professional colleagues who gave their time to travel long distances to participate actively in this meeting and thus generously share their knowledge. Particular thanks go to Professor Arthur Kleinman, Harvard Medical School, for acting as overall chairman of the meeting; to Kathy Iacopini from the Sir Robert Mond Memorial Trust and Maria Eppel from the International Federation of Health Funds for their invaluable support and assistance with the administrative organisation of this meeting; to Pamela Charlton and Gill Nissen from the Publications Unit and Tine Horwitz from the Legal Unit, WHO Regional Office for Europe for their help and guidance with the publication of these proceedings; to Dr John Henderson for his invaluable advice and finally to the British Museum, who, by allowing use of the Egyptian Room for the Reception, enabled delegates to share in the wonders of the Sir Robert Mond Egyptian Collection.

Sponsors

The WHO Regional Office for Europe acknowledges with thanks the contribution made by SmithKline Beecham and Pharmacia & Upjohn to the costs of the meeting, and by Pfizer, in the form of an educational grant, to the cost of publishing the proceedings.

Scope and purpose
of the meeting

This international meeting on unipolar depression was organised by the WHO Office for Quality in Non-Communicable Diseases & Conditions, London, in co-operation with the International Federation of Health Funds, the Harvard School of Medicine and the Sir Robert Mond Memorial Trust. It is the first in a series of formal activities undertaken by the WHO Office in furtherance of its primary remit, to identify centres of proven excellence and through them encourage the development of quality care management programmes for use in central and eastern Europe.

Aim of the meeting

The meeting aimed to address Target 6 of the WHO health for all policy, which deals with improving mental health care in primary, community and secondary care settings. In the United Kingdom it also addressed the National Health Service priorities for mental health.

The objective of the meeting was to increase the understanding of all those involved in the diagnosis and treatment of people with depression of the need for early diagnosis, especially of those with unusual clinical presentations, and of the clinical and financial benefits of prompt intervention with therapeutic courses of appropriate antidepressants. It was hoped that raising awareness would act as a lever for further quality care development in this area. It targeted colleagues working in primary care, policymakers at national, regional and local levels, as well as those involved in health insurance and independent healthcare.

Eminent researchers in the field of unipolar depression from the United States of America, Canada, Australia, France, the Netherlands,

Switzerland, Denmark and the United Kingdom addressed the meeting. The areas they covered included:

- depression as a global public health burden;
- novel methods for the early detection of unipolar depression (WHO (five) Wellbeing Index, Progressor SF36 and others);
- male depression and its potential association with domestic violence, especially during pregnancy;
- problems surrounding the increase in young male suicides;
- economic implications of the clinical condition and of drug therapy;
- problems for diagnosis and treatment in primary care;
- political and social responses to depression;
- somatisation of depression;
- depression and stress;
- implications for industry and the work place.

Time did not allow the inclusion of several lectures. However, as these covered important areas they have been included in these proceedings for ease of reference.

Over twenty different nationalities attended the meeting. Publication of these proceedings will ensure that they are available to many more worldwide.

Ann Dawson MD
Director
WHO Office for Quality in Non-Communicable Diseases & Conditions
London

Opening Session

Welcoming addresses

Can we turn the table on depression?

JO ERIK ASVALL

It is a great pleasure for me to welcome you on behalf of WHO's Regional Office for Europe; a region comprising 51 countries and their 870 million people from Greenland in the west, to the Mediterranean in the south and the Pacific shores of the Russian Federation in the east. I am delighted that this meeting is organised jointly with the International Federation of Health Funds, the Harvard Medical School and the Sir Robert Mond Memorial Trust – together we represent a unique blend of expertise, experience and possibilities for influencing the future, which makes this particular meeting so fascinating. A tremendous *potential* is created when such a key body as the International Federation of Health Funds sits down with WHO and people representing the scientific community, to see how the quality of patients' care can be improved through new principles of disease management. I feel right now that we are not just opening a meeting – *we may well be opening the door to a new development that can be of major benefit to people and healthcare systems everywhere!*

Why should we choose a subject like depression to launch this new initiative? There are several good reasons for this. First, in terms of impact on *people's health and quality of life*, depression takes the biggest toll – a staggering 10% of life years lost to disability for the working population globally; twice as much, for example, as tuberculosis or traffic accidents. Depression is an illness that hits *all* of us – young or old, men or women, in all societies – to a greater or lesser extent throughout our life. It is a major trauma for the individual – but also to family and friends; on average, five other individuals are severely affected by one person's serious depression. Depression also represents a major cost to the healthcare system; when not treated at an early stage, it goes on to cost ten times as

3

much as if not dealt with promptly. The total cost of depression to society through lost productivity, healthcare cost, etc. is difficult to assess precisely – but it surely is high indeed!

Even worse, in its more severe form, depression leads to *suicide*. This tragic outcome is responsible for as much as 15% of deaths in 15–25-year-olds in the European Region, a toll now increasing also among the elderly – especially in the newly independent states.

'Fine,' you may say, 'so depression is a big problem – but what can we *do* about it?' Can we really do anything sensible, practical, effective? Yes, we can – and that is why we are here today! Not only are we here to discuss what technical solutions are now available. More importantly: we are here to discuss whether and how we can bring better health to people if *we*, as organisations, adopt new ways of working – and of *working together*!

Can we do something to prevent depression from occurring in the first place? Yes, but only through very broad, consistent, multisectorial action. It is a well-known fact that depression normally is an expression of an imbalance in the person's personality and the external factors that influence him/her as they proceed through life. Clearly, supporting more strongly programmes that aim at giving children from a tender age healthy values and good life skills to cope with problems in a mature way are an investment in health for the individual's future. Such programmes merit more thought from those that have to pay for the consequences of not ensuring such skills at an early age! Schools can provide an excellent opportunity for teaching such life skills and more imaginative health programmes in such settings – as, for example, in WHO's Health Promoting Schools network. The same applies to the work site; carefully designed health promotion programmes have been shown to both improve health problems and productivity – but how many organisations paying for healthcare are willing to go to the root of the problems and invest in such efforts to prevent the higher expenditure that otherwise invariably follows?

Needless to say, major risk factors for depression are often directly linked to public policies regarding education, labour, housing, social welfare, etc. as they can create conditions that are important contributing factors to depression and suicides. Such issues are closely linked to the many serious problems of today's tough and fast-moving societies that disrupt social networks and create instability and consternation for a rapidly increasing number of the population.

'A bleak picture' you may say and rightly so; *preventing* depression surely remains a formidable and complicated challenge for societies. Why bother then to deal with this health problem? Fortunately, not all things are bleak – on the contrary, some look very encouraging indeed ! In recent years, two major events have happened, events that give us a reason for new optimism, opening up promising ways to improve the situation. These two issues are our ability to identify depression at an early stage, and our possibilities for

4

treating it effectively – both areas where we recently have made very important progress.

Until a short while ago, *our ability to identify serious depression* has, to put it mildly, not been good! On average, only some one in three patients who suffer from serious depression and visit a general practitioner will be identified as having such – the other two patients will leave without that diagnosis. Recently, however, a new tool has been developed by WHO and its collaborating experts – *Well-being 5,** a set of five simple questions to measure the degree of wellbeing that the patient can complete in a couple of minutes. Such a test can identify people who are likely to have depression (the final diagnosis to be confirmed by additional tests). Thus, we now have a *screening test* that is very simple to apply and that more than doubles our ability to identify patients in need of treatment!

Furthermore, we also know more about where there are groups at special risk on which we should focus particular attention. Thus, some more recent studies have revealed that stress and/or *depression related to pregnancy* is probably a much bigger problem than previously realised. It also hits the fathers – not only mothers, as previously thought. No less important, the *effect* of depression on fathers, in a number of cases, can be in the form of *violence against family members* – some studies say as much as 40% of violence and divorce in the home starts in connection with first pregnancies! This being the case, programmes for pregnancy control should now clearly also include screening both parents for depression – an extremely cheap and, in all likelihood, very cost-effective approach. Similarly, such screening should represent a very appropriate tool for use in school health service programmes, in health promotion programmes at the work site, etc. Most important, however, may be its extensive use in primary healthcare settings by *family health physicians and family health nurses*. The latter is a new type of nurse that WHO advocates as the frontline worker for health, working for a restricted number of families, spending much of their time in people's homes so that they can acquire a good knowledge of emerging health problems at an early stage when they are still easy to treat. Funding such family health nurse and family health physician programmes would be sensible for payment organisations that are interested in more comprehensive and cost-effective healthcare solutions.

The second piece of good news is that we are not only able to identify problems at an early stage, but *we are also now able to treat depression much more effectively than before*. I will not go through the whole armamentarium of therapeutic methods now available – from improved drug regimes to better psychological counselling – as these will be dealt with by other speakers. Let me just say that there are pilot projects in the European Region, such as the *Gotland Study*, which indicate that training primary healthcare physicians in better diagnosis and treatment skills for depression can have a major beneficial impact – including a substantial reduction in

---

* WHO (five) Wellbeing Index

suicide. True, the impact has been stronger for women than men, but follow up work is now on the way to see how this can be dealt with.

So we can relax then, in the comforting knowledge that early detection and treatment of depression will now rapidly improve? No, unfortunately not; getting the whole healthcare system to change and adopt the new approaches is, unfortunately, a much more complicated issue! Extensive work carried out by WHO in the last 15 years – as well as other research and development – has clearly shown that *it is not enough to issue information on new and improved methods for the practice to change accordingly.* On the contrary, old traditions die much harder in the healthcare system than we like to think, but, fortunately, new approaches to *quality of care development* have recently been developed – and proven to be effective.

A very simple truth has emerged as perhaps the biggest stumbling block for improving quality of care in clinical practice: *no country* in the world has, at the moment, a system whereby the health outcome of daily clinical practice is followed up, recorded and fed back to the individual provider of that care! Thus, to be brutally honest: *physicians, nurses, physiotherapists, psychologists and other healthcare professionals today work blindfolded.* This is not so because we have failed to give them high ethical standards in their education or because their professional organisations do not place concern for their patients as a top priority. The reason for the current situation is that there are simply no systems designed and operating that consistently record such outcome data and feed them back to the individual providers, permitting them to see their own performance compared to their peers.

The result of this is that we find a large variation in healthcare outcomes among countries, regions within countries, institutions within regions, departments within institutions and among individual healthcare providers – this, in spite of all the professional guidelines and all the international research published monthly through professional journals and now globally available to all healthcare practitioners. There is one positive, *very positive*, fact, however; when individual practitioners do get such information and find out how they perform compared to their peers, they – as a rule – have a very strong incentive for improving their performance.

Today's situation also means that aggregate data of quality of care are not available for management of institutional and population-based levels of care. Our *total healthcare systems are, therefore, performing far below the level of cost-effectiveness that current knowledge and available technology ought to produce.* This crucial, very fundamental observation has now been recognised by all the 51 Member States of WHO's European Region in a major challenge for improvement of healthcare performance in the years ahead. Since 1980, the countries of the European Region have had a common health policy framework to guide health development in every Member State. This policy is systematically updated on the basis of changes in health status and new, scientific development of tools that can improve healthcare, ensure a more healthy environment and support more healthy lifestyles. The latest update, approved by all the countries in September 1998 – *HEALTH 21, Health For All in the 21st Century* – sets clear target strategies and indicators both for mental health and quality of care developments. It highlights health outcome focus as the main challenge to reorient management of clinical practice and public health over the next decades; it stresses the need for strict scientific evidence-based clinical practice and strongly advocates close partnerships.

WHO's Regional Office for Europe has worked consistently with these problems over the last 10–15 years. We have recently set up computer systems that permit individual healthcare practitioners, institutions and countries to feed in their own data to our database in Copenhagen and get immediate feedback on their own performance, compared with the total database of experience available in WHO. This has started with perinatal care (where more than 12 million deliveries are now in our database) and diabetes (where hundreds of thousands of patient data are in the database). These systems use minimum data sets of quality indicators agreed upon after close co-operation with WHO and leading professional organisations in Europe. We are now ready to start on mental health, where depression will be the first area; indicators are already available.

Through our networks, WHO has close links to the professional organisations, to every Ministry of Health in the European Region and also to a number of patient organisations that are crucial partners in this work – work that requires efforts from many sources if it is to be the powerful, broad and consistent movement that it must become.

However, we have one major problem at this stage and that is the co-operation of the healthcare payment organisations! *You, the insurance companies of the world that are represented here today, can be a tremendous force to speed up this development*, making it one that reaches out to every healthcare provider in every country or area where you are working. If you require key quality data to be included in your payment systems – with the necessary confidentiality protection – you can have a major influence on the health information systems that are used in daily practice and, thus, help a rapid change to a new culture of working.

Why should you do so? First, an important reason is that *you would help your own clients to get much better care* – and better health for the money they pay you. Could you want a better challenge for your work than to help millions of people in such a fundamental way? Second, you would also *provide a direct economic bonus for yourself*, since the improved care that follows from the outcome focus will, in the large majority of cases, also mean a much more cost-effective use of resources. Thus, a person with diabetes for whom you are responsible, will cost you fifteen times less in annual expenditure when she or he has well-regulated diabetes than one who does not; at least 95% of patients should be able to achieve that level

7

of disease management – as opposed to one-third in today's practice! In short: from being just a *payer* you should become a clearly focused *player* for improved healthcare!

So that is why we meet here – WHO and the representatives of the healthcare payers. We stand at the threshold of a new millennium, but we also stand at a much more important threshold where we can suddenly see that we can manage the whole healthcare system to much higher quality and much better cost-effectiveness. This we can do through quite simple means, using approaches that are already in our hands, that are cheap, feasible, acceptable and tested. Today, WHO reaches out a hand to all of you to work closer together to make this vision become a reality! *Will you grasp it?*

Player and payer: the role of health insurers in improving healthcare provision for people with depression

TOM SACKVILLE

When the opportunity arose in early 1999 to co-organise an international meeting with the WHO Regional Office for Europe, it soon became clear that among possible topics, depression would be a strong candidate. Not least because, of all the non-communicable diseases, the World Health Organization has identified depression as a key area for development. Most of us know someone who is or has been a sufferer and trends indicate that it will be one of the most serious sources of disability in the future, with over 300 million sufferers worldwide by the year 2020. Meanwhile, it is very clear that there is a lack of understanding of the human and economic cost of depression, the connection with the numbers of people who commit or attempt suicide as a direct result, and the increasing availability of effective treatment.

This attitude forms part of a wider set of prejudices about mental illness: while people do not mind discussing serious and fatal conditions such as cancer and heart disease, they steer clear of mental illness. Depression, among those who have not experienced it first hand or in someone close to them, is more likely to be referred to in humorous terms than as a serious threat to public health.

The problem also exists among clinicians, many of whom are unaware of the seriousness of the disease and its close links to other conditions, or have failed to recognise the urgent need to educate themselves about how to diagnose and treat it.

As this meeting demonstrates, there are huge variations in response to depression. At primary care level, some general practitioners will fail to treat effectively, some will rely on non-pharmaceutical intervention or prescribe subtherapeutic doses, while others are fully aware of the latest drugs and their appropriate use. Even among recognised experts on depression, disagreement persists as to whether the latest generation of drugs give the best response.

Whether the payer concerned is governmental or part of the independent sector, the same pressures apply. Media commentators, politicians, consumer organisations and other opinion formers concentrate on the shortcomings of their health services in relation to the more easily understood serious conditions such as cancer and coronary heart disease.

In the United Kingdom, there is little doubt that waiting times for hip replacements and other non-emergency surgery occupy a much more prominent place in the public perception of health than any form of mental illness. If people were fully aware of the number of lives, of both depression sufferers and their families, that are scarred as a result of lack of effective treatment, there would be outrage.

My organisation, the International Federation of Health Funds, is a leading international network of health insurers with a group of substantial healthcare payers in over 20 countries. It clearly has a strong interest in improving its response to depression. WHO, as well as members of the IFHF, see the need for payers to become more proactive in this area by becoming players as well as payers. Many of them have travelled great distances to be here today, some as speakers but most as delegates. Our commitment to continue to help improve care for people with depression globally is thus evident. Members realise that it is in everybody's interest for the payers to take a more proactive role, it makes sense, both financially and in terms of member satisfaction in the future. That is why so many are here today, not only to learn more about the condition but also to identify various ways of linking with healthcare providers and other partners to ensure a better service for the future.

As we enter the twenty-first century and the internet age, the 'informed patient' will become a major factor in clinical practice. The new breed of consumer of health service will not accept second best, and will increasingly challenge clinicians or health payers over the quality and effectiveness of treatment decisions. Both these groups will need to be sure they are armed with evidence-based information on best practice.

This meeting has the benefit of an impressive array of internationally recognised experts on depression, who will make an important contribution to this process. I would like to express my thanks to them, to our sponsors, to all those involved at the World Health Organization and the Sir Robert Mond Trust for their efforts in making all this possible.

A global view of depression from an anthropological perspective

ARTHUR KLEINMAN and ALEX COHEN

The reason to take a global view of depression, an anthropologist's perspective, is that the cross-cultural evidence stands as a challenge to Euro-American perceptions of this condition. Indeed, we maintain that consideration of the cross-cultural evidence is necessary if we expect to move toward a science of depression. What kind of a science could it be that restricts analysis to data from Europe and North America where less than 20% of the world's population resides?

First, what do we know?

- The symptoms of the disease depression include: feelings of dysphoria, hopelessness, fatigue, somatic complaints such as headache and back pain, sleep disruptions, significant loss of weight, functional and social disability, and thoughts of death.
- Rates of depression, like all other health conditions, are strongly associated with socioeconomic status – higher prevalence rates are found among the poor. (Yet, unlike other medical fields, psychiatry tends to ignore social class.)[1,2]
- Worldwide, hundreds of millions of people suffer from depression. According to the most recent data (1998), unipolar major depression, accounts for 4.2% of the world's total burden of disease as measured by Disability Adjusted Life Years (DALYs). This made it the fifth leading cause of disability behind acute lower respiratory infections (6.0%), perinatal conditions (5.8%), diarrhoeal diseases (5.3%), and HIV/AIDS (5.1%).[3]
- Women, worldwide, have rates of depression that are two to three times higher than the rates found among men.

11

- If one looks at persons 15–44 years, a particularly active and productive age group, depression accounted for more than 10% of all DALYs and was the single leading cause of disease burden in the world in 1990 both in high- and in low- and middle-income countries alike.[4]
- Epidemiological research has also demonstrated that between 10% and 25% of attenders in primary care settings – *globally* – are suffering from a mental disorder, most frequently depression and mixed depression/anxiety. Yet, few are diagnosed as such, fewer still receive treatment of any kind, and only a tiny minority of those in need are fortunate enough to be offered appropriate care.[5]
- Our perceptions of depression cross-culturally have changed remarkably. Fifty years ago, for example, there was a widespread belief that Africans did not suffer from depression.[6] This racist notion has been refuted by epidemiological research, which demonstrated that the peoples of subSaharan Africa, if anything, suffer from *higher* rates of depression than European and North American populations.[7, 8]

Yet, as much as we know, the vast majority of the evidence comes from patient populations in North America and Europe. Hence, there is a distortion in the politics of science that follows the political economy of the world and even classical colonialism in some regard. Just consider what happens if we take the data from the developing world where the vast majority of the patients who have depression live. Somatic complaints, not feelings of sadness and loss, are the symptom most commonly reported.[9] Epidemiological surveys in China reveal relatively low rates of depression (at least five times less than those in North America),[10] yet China has relatively high rates of suicide – this runs counter to the notion in Western psychiatry that most suicides are associated with depression.[11] Furthermore, data from the developing world demonstrate the need to consider the social roots of depression. The work of Broadhead and Abas[7] shows the role of traumatic life events, grief, and insoluble problems arising from personal crises in producing high rates of depression among women in Zimbabwe. Other studies from Asia and Africa show the strong relationship between poverty, illiteracy and gender, on one hand, and high rates of depression, on the other.[12-15] There is also extensive evidence concerning the deleterious effects of dislocation and violence on mental health. In migrant populations and in social settings of breakdown, depression clusters together with substance abuse, abuse of women and children, and other related forms of violence.[1] And there is fascinating work on cultural customs that suggest they can protect women against postpartum depression, as has been reported for Fiji.[16]

More generally, we will only achieve a better understanding of depression, by focusing our attention on several key social realities. First, depression is a culturally patterned disorder in that the symptoms and course of the disorder display considerable variation cross-culturally.[9,17] It is also true that depression follows a social course of disease.[1,2] The economics of treatment (i.e. who has access to care?) and social environments (e.g. extreme poverty, gender inequities, violence, and dislocation) have a significant influence on the rates and outcomes of depression. Finally, we must not assume that interventions that have proved efficacious in the West, are equally successful elsewhere. This is obviously the case for various modes of psychotherapy, but it is also true for psychopharmacological interventions. There are significant cross-ethnic and cross-national differences in responses to virtually all psychotropic medications, and optimal dosing practices and side-effect profiles vary significantly among different populations.[18]

With this evidence about social influence on depression, it is indeed curious that academic psychiatry has turned so overwhelmingly to the investigation of the biological roots of depression. We will not argue that neurobiological research must be abandoned, or even that it should not be pursued vigorously, but we do find it troubling that psychiatry seems to be turning away from other areas of investigation. To draw two analogies. Would it have been better if John Snow had confined himself to finding the bacillus that causes cholera rather than identifying the water source that was responsible for the cholera epidemic in London? Can we discount the work of Ignaz Semmelweis because, rather than finding either bacteriological cause or cure, he suggested that mortality from childbed fever could be reduced if doctors washed their hands after examining each patient? Snow and Semmelweis demonstrated that understanding the social roots of cholera and puerperal fever – even in the absence of a biological understanding of their aetiologies – was enormously important. Psychiatry must do the same.

Furthermore, there is now abundant evidence that shows the enormous impact of the social world on biology.[19-22] We need to move away from the notion that biology is somehow immutably universal and completely remote to the social world. That is not the view of biologists. Rather, it is a misunderstanding that has dominated biological psychiatry. Most biologists regard biology as the great source of variation.[23] Most psychiatrists regard biology as the great source of similarity. Neurobiologists envision the brain as neural processes open to influence from the social world; neural networks responding to social networks.[24] Would that more biological psychiatrists saw genes in their contexts – bodily and social – in the same interactive way. Perhaps it is an issue of the chronic (and to some extent understandable) sensitivity of psychiatrists to past attacks that challenged a biomedical approach to mental illness and also their defensiveness that, in spite of much interesting research data, the biological mechanisms in depression and schizophrenia are still unknown. Nevertheless, the psychiatric understanding of biology is a problem, and it is why the global perspective on depression is so vitally important. Cross-cultural variation, higher rates of disorder among the poorest 20% of the world's population, the large gender gap, and the social cluster of disorders must become the very bases of psychiatric research, rather than a mere annoyance, 'noise' in statistical analyses, that must be controlled. Biology and culture come together in sociosomatic processes that need to become the focus of cross-disciplinary research.[25]

As much as we know about depression, it is remarkable that we know more about the illness experiences (narratives of suffering and coping) of patients with diabetes, heart disease, or cancer than we know about patients who suffer from depression. If we consider the developing world, we know almost nothing about the everyday lived experiences of people with depression. To truly understand depression, to move toward developing a valid psychiatric research agenda, we must begin with local phenomenology, with the way people experience their lives, with their experiences of dysphoria, pain, loss of hope, and other core symptoms, and then consider what people do about those experiences: from whom do they seek treatment; what kinds of treatment do they get; and how do they evaluate the outcome?

A better understanding of the illness experiences of persons with depression will also be useful in avoiding the conflation of affect and disease. While it is true that individuals in the midst of grief or in the end stages of life may present symptoms of sadness or feelings of loss, we must be careful not to medicalise suffering. That these individuals might benefit from psychopharmacological or psychotherapeutic interventions does not mean we can ignore the realities with which they are trying to cope. Similarly, while a woman in Zimbabwe or Goa might benefit from treatment for depression, one must also attend to the conditions (e.g. poverty, gender inequities and illiteracy) that are associated with her depression. Indeed, those conditions will also affect access and adherence to treatment. This is how epidemiologists and clinicians understand multidrug-resistant tuberculosis and HIV/AIDS and most other biomedical disorders, and it is how we need to consider depression.

Everywhere in the world, depression represents a major source of the burden of disease. As the developing world continues to make the epidemiological transition, as the proportion of morbidity and mortality from non-communicable diseases begins to exceed that from infectious diseases, the relative burden of depression will increase. To meet that challenge, psychiatry must expand its scope of interests – making them more international, more cross-cultural, more social – so that it will be able to make a significant contribution to the recognition and treatment of depression in all of its manifestations.

References

1. Desjarlais R, Eisenberg L, Good B, Kleinman A. *World Mental Health: problems and priorities in low-income countries.* New York: Oxford University Press, 1995.
2. World Health Organization. *The World Health Report 1995: bridging the gaps.* Geneva: World Health Organization, 1995.

3. World Health Organization. *World Health Report 1999: making a difference.* Geneva: World Health Organization, 1999.
4. Murray CJL, Lopez AD., eds *The Global Burden of Disease.* Cambridge, MA: Harvard University Press, 1996.
5. Üstün T, Sartorius N. *Mental illness in general healthcare: an international study.* Chichester: John Wiley, 1995.
6. Carothers JC. *The African Mind in Health and Disease: a study in ethnopsychiatry.* Geneva: World Health Organization, 1953.
7. Broadhead J, Abas M. Life events, difficulties and depression among women in an urban setting in Zimbabwe. *Psychological Med* 1998;**28**:29–38.
8. Orley J, Wing JK. Psychiatric disorders in two African villages. *Arch Gen Psychiatry* 1979;**36**:513–20.
9. Kleinman AM. *Rethinking Psychiatry: from cultural category to personal experience.* New York: Free Press, 1988.
10. Kleinman A. China: the epidemiology of mental illness. *Br J Psychiatry* 1996;**169**:129–30.
11. Phillips M, Liu H, Zhang Y. Suicide and social change in China. *Culture, Med Psychiatry* 1999;**23**:25–50.
12. Gureje O, Omigbodun OO. Children with mental disorders in primary care: functional status and risk factors. *Acta Psychiatr Scand* 1995;**92**:310–4.
13. Patel V, Pereira J, Coutinho L, Fernandes R. Poverty, psychological disorder and disability in primary care attenders in Goa, India. *Br J Psychiatry* 1998;**172**:533–6.
14. Patel V, Todd C, Winston M et al. Common mental disorders in primary care in Harare, Zimbabwe: associations and risk factors. *Br J Psychiatry* 1997;**171**:60–4.
15. Tafari S, Aboud FE, Larson CP. Determinants of mental illness in a rural Ethiopian adult population. *Social Sci Med* 1991;**32**:197–201.
16. Becker AE. Postpartum illness in Fiji: a sociosomatic perspective. *Psychosom Med* 1998;**60**:431–8.
17. Manson SM. Culture and major depression: current challenges in the diagnosis of mood disorders. *Psychiatr Clin North America* 1995;**18**:487–501.
18. Lin K-M, Anderson D, Poland RE. Ethnicity and psychopharmacology. *Psychiatr Clin North America* 1995;**18**:635–47.
19. Ellison PT. Reproductive ecology and 'local biology' [Paper presented at the panel 'Bridging the cultural and biological divide']. Annual meeting, American Anthropological Association, San Francisco, 20 November, 1996.
20. Ellison PT. Reproductive ecology and reproductive cancers. In: Panter-Brick C, Worthman CM, eds. *Hormones, Health, and Behavior: a socio-ecological and lifespan perspective.* Cambridge, MA: Cambridge University Press, 1999: 184–203.
21. Lewontin R. *Human Diversity.* New York: Scientific American Library, 1995.
22. Ramachandran VS, Blakeslee S. *Phantoms in the Brain: probing the mysteries of the human mind.* New York: William Morrow, 1998.
23. Mayr E. *The Growth of Biological Thought: diversity, evolution, and inheritance.* Cambridge, MA: Belknap Press of Harvard University Press, 1982.
24. Eisenberg L. The social construction of the human brain. *Am J Psychiatry* 1995;**152**:1563–9.
25. Kleinman A, Becker AE. 'Sociosomatics': the contributions of anthropology to psychosomatic medicine. *Psychosom Med* 1998;**60**:389–93.

Opening Address

Unipolar postnatal depression – at what cost?

JOHN COX

I was delighted to accept the invitation to give an opening address at this important conference for reasons that were corporate, as an endorsement by the Royal College of Psychiatrists of the meeting theme, and individual, as I have been a researcher in this field for almost three decades.

For this meeting to focus particularly on unipolar depression was indeed an imaginative and timely step as these common disorders are so often overlooked and yet are a major family and economic burden. I am not sure, however, if such depression is a timebomb waiting to explode because it had already exploded. The World Health Organization (1990) as well as national governments are at last recognising that depression not only accounts for 10% of the total burden of disease but that neuropsychiatric problems cause up to 30% of Disability Adjusted Life Years.

Thus unipolar postnatal depression, for example, affects at least 1 in 10 women, and may have an immediate adverse effect on the mother–infant relationship, and on the economic prosperity of the family. Furthermore, such depressive illnesses are often neglected by health service planners because they may not appear to be so conspicuously disabling as schizophrenia or as a severe obsessive–compulsive disorder. Depressive sufferers do not intercept London commuters on their way to work and yet 1 in 15 of these commuters are likely themselves to be suffering from a depression that could be effectively treated.

It is at last recognised by the [UK] Department of Health in its recent *Mental Health National Service Framework for Adults of Working Age*[1] that depression is indeed a severe mental illness because of its duration, personal distress, family burden and economic cost. This framework includes a well-referenced section on postnatal depression, and

19

recommends the development of clinical practice guidelines for referral from primary to secondary care services.

My earlier research interest in perinatal psychiatry was first triggered by the work of Pitt[2] who published in 1968 his seminal paper on postnatal depression in which he referred to postnatal depression as 'atypical'. Three hundred and five women living in the East End of London who attended an antenatal clinic were followed to the puerperium when 10.8% were found to have become depressed after delivery. Pitt found that over a third of these women remained depressed when contacted 12 months later; a self-report questionnaire was developed for this study to measure the change in depression between the last trimester of pregnancy and six weeks' postpartum.

In Uganda I completed what was I believe the first controlled prospective study of postnatal depression[3] and could confirm not just that depression was a common mood disorder in a semirural African population (which was contested at that time) but that 10% of women three months' postpartum had been continuously depressed since delivery. For a third, their day-to-day work, including the carrying of water and growing food, was noticeably impaired. This study together with my later studies in Edinburgh provided the stimulus to develop a ten-item Edinburgh Postnatal Depression Scale (EPDS)[4] to be administered by health professionals at or about the six week postnatal visit. The EPDS has been translated into over 12 languages, is used in research as a first-stage screening procedure and is now used to assist the primary and secondary prevention of depression. Because of this work abroad I have remained particularly interested in the effect of culture on the presentation and classification of depressive disorders and was sensitised especially to the need for a transcultural perspective if a full understanding of postnatal depression was to be obtained.

The auspices of this meeting, which included the Harvard Medical School and Arthur Kleinman's imprimatur, was a further realisation that our meeting could be strategic and influence national governments as well as those working in international organisations.

The tendency for mood disorder research units to 'overlook' depression postpartum is an unfortunate limitation of much research at the present time; a neglect that may be explained by the nosological muddle of the postnatal mood disorders as well as by an understanding that postnatal depression requires an assessment of biological and sociological triggering factors – it is necessary, therefore, to bridge two research methodologies and conceptual frameworks. The full recognition of the explanatory power of a childbirth-linked mood disorder may assist in understanding the reasons for the higher rates of depression in women than men and could encourage further consideration of the causes of Dysthymia. Some international studies have overlooked recording the onset of depression in relation to childbirth and parity may not have been noted.

In the UK National Psychiatric Morbidity Survey (1998)[5], for example, which found almost twice the rate of depression and anxiety in women of childbearing age, whether the women were pregnant or recently delivered were not, alas, recorded. Yet postnatal depression research findings suggest that a possible explanation for the increased rate of depression in this age group is depression triggered or exacerbated within eight weeks following childbirth.

In the controlled study we carried out in 1993 in North Staffordshire, the prevalence of postpartum depression at three months was 13%; a similar frequency to the non-childbearing controls.[6] Yet a threefold increased onset rate of depression in the first five weeks' postpartum was found when compared to the equivalent time period for controls.

The social burden on families can be illustrated by the comments of carers (mostly by husbands)[7] (see Box 1). These findings suggest that the economic effect of such depression on employment may be considerable.

Counsellors in RELATE describe the frequency with which they are consulted by depressed couples after childbirth, and that marital breakdown and divorce occur at that time (an association reported earlier

---

Box 1   Impact of postnatal depression on the family: the verbatim experience of carers (mostly husbands)

'We don't like to see her so low and depressed.'

'I feel fed up as I don't like to see her upset.'

'I want to help her, but I don't know how.'

'This has put a lot of stress on both of us.'

'She makes you feel depressed.'

'I am glad to see that someone realises that men are affected as well. All treatments are geared towards mothers – fathers are affected too.'

'No help or acknowledgement that the father is affected by postnatal depression as well as the mother.'

'It's like having two babies, all assistance is aimed at the mother. Fathers need help too.'

'Afraid of saying something out of turn in case of causing an argument.'

'She's very touchy.'

'Flares up at the slightest thing causing arguments.'

'I don't know how to approach her because of her moods.'

---

by Dominian8 in his influential book on marital breakdown). Almost all studies in the field of postnatal depression find an association between postnatal depression and marital difficulty and hassle.

Depression has an immediate effect on the mother–infant relationship, and at 18 months there may be insecure attachment when compared with the children of non-depressed mothers; at five years, cognitive impairment, particularly in boys, has also been found.[9] Postnatal depression can be prevented by identifying a high-risk group of women at the booking-in clinic; e.g. women with a past or family history of mental disorder and an unwanted baby, especially where there is an unsupportive partner.

The *Confidential Inquiry into Maternal Deaths in the United Kingdom*[10] found that the frequency of death through suicide was of a similar magnitude to women dying from toxaemia during pregnancy. This report made, therefore, specific recommendations to screen for postnatal depression in the community and to identify high-risk women at the booking-in clinic.

The increased frequency of depression when family structures are changing, is indeed a timebomb the effects of which may only be fully discovered in the next generation when infants born into these distressed families become disadvantaged and when they themselves become parents.

Our society may therefore have to decide in what way to adjust to new patterns of parenthood. If existing patterns of family life are to be maintained then specific mental health services structured to provide prevention and therapeutic strategies for parents with perinatal mood disorder are quite indispensable.

References

1. *Mental Health National Service Framework for Adults of Working Age*. London: Department of Health, 1999.
2. Pitt B. 'Atypical' depression following childbirth. *Br J Psychiatry* 1968;**114**:1325–35.
3. Cox JL. Postnatal depression: a comparison of African and Scottish women. *Social Psychiatry* 1983;**18**:25–8.
4. Cox JL, Holden JM, Sagovsky R. Detection of postnatal depression; development of the Edinburgh Postnatal Depression Scale. *Br J Psychiatry* 1987;**150**:782–6.
5. Meltzer H, Gill B, Pettigrew M The prevalence of psychiatric morbidity among adults aged 16–64, living in private households in Great Britain. *OPCS Surveys of Psychiatric Morbidity in Great Britain, Bulletin no. 1*. London: Office of Population Censuses and Surveys.
6. Cox JL. Murray D, Chapman G. A controlled study of the onset duration and prevalence of postnatal depression. *Br J Psychiatry* 1993;**163**:27–31.
7. Boath EH, Pryce AJ, Cox JL. Postnatal depression: the impact on the family. *J Reprod Infant Psychol* 1998;**16**:199–203.
8. Dominian J. *Marital Breakdown*. London: Penguin Books, 1968.
9. Sharp D, Hay DF, Pawlby S *et al*. The impact of postnatal depression on boys' intellectual development. *J Child Psychol Psychiatry* 1995;**36**:1315.
10. *Confidential Enquiry into Maternal Deaths in the United Kingdom 1994–1996*. London: HMSO.

Setting the Scene
Overview

This opening section provides important background information commencing with an historical review of the treatment of depression over the past 300 years, from the patient's and the doctor's perspectives. This extremely informative article will be of interest not only to doctors but also to those with an interest in social and medical history. The following two articles give global views of depression but from slightly different perspectives. The first addresses cost effectiveness and possible ways of reducing the burden. The second reviews depression over the past 50 years, tracing the introduction of the newer forms of drug therapy.

The problem of depression in the elderly is next discussed. Currently the over-65-year-olds account for 29% of the population; by 2020 this will have risen to over 30%. Managing the age-related needs of an unprecedentedly large and rapidly growing aged population will be one of the key public health challenges of the next 50 years. Older people are prone to depression, especially those who live communally, who are six to ten times more likely to suffer from depression than those who live alone. Treatment in this group can be difficult. Consideration is also given to whether or not late-onset depression differs in any way to early-onset depression.

Next discussed is the problem of somatisation, which is the expression of psychological distress through physical symptoms, and accounts for a substantial proportion of undiagnosed psychiatric morbidity in primary care. Approximately 80% of primary care attenders present with somatic symptoms. Failure to diagnose the underlying cause for these symptoms can be quite costly, especially to the patient. Men and women express their depression in different ways. Men tend to suppress their feelings during the early stages but as the condition progresses pent-up feelings can be released resulting in aggressive behaviour especially towards the partner. It is therefore important to have tools that can easily identify depression, especially masked or covert depression. The problem of male depression, stress and aggression are picked up in the next two articles. The various methods for quick and easy identification of depression, using the WHO (five)WellBeing Index are discussed in one of these articles, and the problems of inappropriate medication and the value of continuous educative programmes for general practitioners are discussed in the other article (Gotland Study).

Historical review of diagnosis and treatment of depression

EDWARD SHORTER

Depression has passed from being a rather obscure illness called 'melancholia' mainly seen in asylums, to the number one source of clinical disability in the world.[1] This is a familiar trajectory for psychiatric illnesses: from obscurity to epidemic status. Obsessive–compulsive disorder, panic and traumatic stress have all experienced similar inflations in their popularity. How has depression become the number one chronic illness in the world? Is this a true finding? And, above all, what can we do about it?

In charting the history of depression we must keep in mind that there are two narratives: the doctor's and the patient's. The doctor's narrative is the tale of formal diagnosis and treatment, and how they have changed over the last two centuries, originating with the diagnosis of melancholia that goes back to the Ancients.[2] The patient's narrative concerns what is often dismissively referred to as 'medical folklore': how average people have conceived dysphoria, and how their urgings have influenced the nature of medical help provided to them. George Bernard Shaw's 1911 warning in the preface to his play *The Doctor's Dilemma* remains as true for the doctor–patient relationship today as for the Edwardians: '[Doctors] must believe, on the whole, what their patients believe, just as they must wear the sort of hat their patients wear... When the patient has a prejudice the doctor must either keep it in countenance or lose his patient.'[3] In other words, physicians must more or less do what their patients expect of them.

Physicians have always recognised the core of melancholia in the concept of depression: patients who cried all the time, had a diminished sense of self-worth, and viewed their lives as hopeless. Oxford's Robert Burton, though a non-physician, is thought of as originating the modern medical doctrine of depression. In 1621 he versified of melancholia:[4]

When I lie waking all alone,
Recounting what I have ill done,
My thoughts on me then tyrannise,
Fear and sorrow me surprise,
Whether I tarry still or go,
Methinks the time moves very slow,
All my griefs to this are jolly,
Naught so sad as Melancholy.

Parisian psychiatrist Philippe Pinel, generally regarded as the founder of modern psychiatry, described 'mélancholie' in 1801 as 'the most pusilanimous dejection, a profound consternation or even despair'. He saw the symptoms as belonging to 'a melancholic constitution', a kind of disposition with which one was born. For him, it characterised the English.[5]

Physicians gave such diagnoses as hypochondria to other forms of depression, such as the somatised version with its predominance of aches and pains. Seen as 'hysteria,' somatisation was not really recognised as having much in common with mood disorders. Such psychosomatic symptoms certainly did not constitute, for the physicians of the day, 'depressive-equivalents'. Thus at their point of departure in the narrative, the doctors recognised depression only in the relatively restrictive form of melancholia.

Yet the patients have a narrative too, and in their narrative dysphoria, dejection and self-debasement have always been recognised. It is of interest that, in England, the patients often selected the term 'depression' for symptoms that the doctors of the time deemed 'melancholia.' Thus Fanny Burney, a young aristocratic woman of the late-eighteenth century, brushed often against the illness. It was studded throughout her family tree. In 1792, after a family visit she wrote in her diary of her father: 'I found ... my dear Father rather worse than better, and lower and more depressed about himself than ever. To see him dejected is, of all sights, to me the most melancholy.' A month later she referred to 'my father's continued illness and depression.'[6]

In the patient's world, the treatment of 'depression' involved spas, mineral waters, and rest much more than did the doctors' concept of treatment, which tended to invoke such medications as hellebore (*Veratrum viride*). It was common for the relatives of a depressed individual to pack the patient off on an ocean voyage or to a spa such as Baden-Baden with the cheery advice that all the afflicted member needed was 'a change of scenery,' and that with the many diversions of spa life he or she would be feeling better in no time. Yet 'depression' in the patient's world before 1900 was not a frequent category, and patients preferred to attribute symptoms to their 'nerves' in such expressions as 'a nervous breakdown', or 'nervous exhaustion', neither of which has ever constituted a real medical diagnosis.

The nineteenth century saw a huge expansion of medical diagnoses for dysphoria. In 1869, George Beard coined the term 'neurasthenia', the diagnostic criteria for which were so broad that it encompassed everything from loss of a night's sleep to full-bore psychosis. In the world of medical practice, however, the core symptoms of neurasthenia soon became coterminous with those of depression, centring on mood, energy, and vegetative functions.[7] 'Hysteria' was the depression-equivalent diagnosis for women, although its core symptoms tended to centre more on bodily function than mood. And Pierre Janet's 'psychasthenia' served nicely for mood disorders in both sexes.

Yet the rule is that doctors like to diagnose what they are able to treat. As the illness depression grew more treatable, the diagnostic term 'depression' came increasingly to replace melancholia within medicine. The first real psychopharmacological treatment of depression to supplant hellebore was the opium cure, popularised in the nineteenth century by the Engelken family, a psychiatric dynasty that owned a private nervous clinic near Bremen. It was after the 1840s that the family began to publicise the recipe of what had previously been their 'secret powder'.[8] In the 1860s 'depression' begins to appear as a diagnostic category in the medical dictionaries.[9]

The treatment of depression took a massive leap forward in 1938 with the introduction of ECT, electroconvulsive therapy, by Ugo Cerletti, the professor of psychiatry in Rome. With ECT, melancholic depression became eminently treatable, and the whole concept of treating depression became medically more appealing than traditional 'melancholia' had been, with its aura of hopelessness, grief, and impending suicide. In 1952, DSM-I (as it was later called), the first edition of the DSM series of the American Psychiatric Association, gave prominent play to 'depressive reactions', which the manual rather bizarrely insisted were symptoms of underlying efforts to deal with anxiety.[10] Depression had now become a familiar diagnosis within psychiatry.

Yet there is a large distance between familiar and epidemic. To understand the almost epidemic status that depression has achieved today, we must consider developments in both the doctor's and the patient's narratives. The introduction of the antidepressants in 1958 was of epochal significance in the recognition of depression. Now that depression was pharmacologically treatable, its diagnosis began to rise in frequency.[11] To be sure, the introduction of the benzodiazepines in 1960 placed the diagnosis 'anxiety' in centre stage for the next two decades. Yet there is no doubt that, as American psychiatry began to distance itself from psychoanalysis – with its announced indifference to precise diagnosis – such diagnoses as depression gained in currency. DSM-III, introduced in 1980, offered a plethora of possibilities for making the depression diagnosis. Thomas Ban has calculated that DSM-IV (1994) provides 608 variations for diagnosing depression.[12]

The introduction of the selective serotonin-reuptake inhibitors (SSRIs) – first by Astra Pharmaceuticals in the form of zimelidine (Zelmid) in 1982, then as Eli-Lilly's fluoxetine (Prozac) in 1987 – gave the diagnosis of depression yet another great push forward. In 1985, 'depressive disorders' had represented only 29.5% of all diagnoses given by American psychiatrists in private practice. By 1995, the figure had grown to 46.8%.[13] Almost half of all American psychiatric patients were said to be depressed. Clearly, American psychiatrists liked to diagnose what they were able to treat, and by 1995 they deemed themselves able to treat depression. (Anxiety disorders, by contrast, had receded from 17.7% of all diagnoses to 11.1%.)

Healy sees the decision to give the SSRIs prescription-only status as crucial in their conquest of the depression market. In effect, not only was a drug-class being marketed but a 'lesion' concept of depressive illness as well, the lesion being a monoamine deficiency. Healy writes: 'Retrospectively, then it should be no surprise that the restriction of sales to a disease market should have been associated with an apparent increase in the amount of disease in the community.'[14]

But there is more to the story. The practice of psychiatry does not exist in a vacuum, and this epidemic growth of the depression diagnosis would probably not have occurred without pressure from the patient's world. It had been the patients who introduced the term 'depression' in the eighteenth century. The phrase slumbered on across the years, alongside such hardy perennials as 'nerves' and 'the blues'. Then after the 1950s, as a result of the success of the first generation of tricyclic antidepressants, 'depression' began to undergo a revival among patients.

The number of references to depression and its therapy in American magazines grew dramatically between 1950 and the 1990s, up from zero in 1950 to 70 in 1995 (although the highpoint, in this sampling of five-year intervals, was 1985, with 84 articles) (Table 1).

The stage was thus set for the 'Prozac craze' that commenced in the 1990s. In the world of medical folklore, people increasingly defined their dysphoria in terms of depression. And physicians had popular new antidepressants ready to hand in the form of the SSRIs (in contrast to the first generation of antidepressants that made patients feel leaden and caused them to gain weight). Such was the popularity of Prozac in the United States that it started to become a street drug, sold outside pharmacies.

It was this reality of the SSRIs also treating 'unhappiness' that lent them their virtual cult status in the patient's world. (In addition to a large amount of anecdotal evidence that the SSRIs improve unhappiness, Knutson and fellow researchers found that, in a sample group of normal human volunteers, 'SSRI administration reduced negative affect relative to placebo.'[15]) This cult status, in turn, increased pressure upon psychiatrists to prescribe them.[16] Because the indication 'unhappiness' was seen disapprovingly by the insurance companies, the wings of the 'depression' diagnosis unfolded ever more. For humanitarian and commercial reasons, therefore, American psychiatry found the pressure to conflate unhappiness with 'depression' virtually irresistible.

Table 1 Frequency of articles on 'depression' in American magazines, five-year intervals, 1950–95

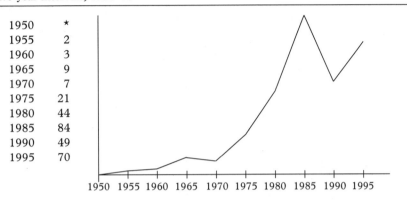

Year	Count
1950	*
1955	2
1960	3
1965	9
1970	7
1975	21
1980	44
1985	84
1990	49
1995	70

*In 1950 there were a few articles on mental hygiene, nervous breakdowns, nervousness and anxiety.

What future prospects do these reflections give rise to? First of all, when we discuss the psychopharmacology of depression, what we may really have in mind is the psychopharmacology of unhappiness. Unhappiness, as we know, responds readily – if not durably – to ethanol. It certainly responds to such street drugs as cocaine. And it responds, as a generation of users can now testify, to the SSRIs. Thus, psychiatry is able to treat unhappiness.

But we are gathered together to discuss the worldwide burden of depression, not that of unhappiness, the latter having structural and happenstance components. We therefore do well to keep in mind:

- That there is indeed an enormous worldwide burden of unhappiness.
- That some of this unhappiness is the result of psychiatric illness.
- Finally, that some of this illness is clinical depression.

A formulation of this nature helps us to prevent psychiatric imperialism, meaning the conversion of all human problems into 'illness.' It also gives us a logic for holding the pharmaceutical industry at arm's length. SSRIs make everybody feel good. They are in fact for many a kind of magic pill for unhappiness caused by the structure of their lives. But it is not the job of psychiatry to lend the lustre of science to this kind of folkloric self-medication that is driven forward by commercial interests.

One remembers that physicians love to diagnose what they can treat. They can now treat depression successfully, but that does not automatically mean that a majority of their patients are depressed. Depression is indeed a common illness. But the irony is that the more successful the treatment, the commoner it becomes.

References

1. Murray CJL, Lopez AD, eds. *The Global Burden of Disease*, p. 236. Cambridge, MA: Harvard University Press, 1996.
2. Jackson SW. *Melancholia and Depression from Hippocratic Times to Modern Times*. New Haven, CT: Yale University Press, 1986.
3. Shaw GB. *The Doctor's Dilemma*, p.67. Harmondsworth: Penguin, 1946.
4. Burton R. *The Anatomy of Melancholy*, p.8. New York: Tudor, 1948.
5. Pinel P. *Traité Médico-philosophique sur l'Aliénation Mentale, ou la Manie*. 2nd edn, pp.39, 166. Paris: Brosson, 1809.
6. Burney F. *The Journals and Letters of Fanny Burney (Madame D'Arblay)*, vol 1, pp.115, 132. Oxford: Clarendon Press, 1972.
7. Wessely S. Old wine in new bottles: neurasthenia and 'ME'. *Psychol Med* 1990;**20**:35–53.
8. Schmitz H. Die Opiumbehandlung bei Geisteskrankheiten insbesondere bei Melancholie, ihre Geschichte, ihr heutiger Stand und eigene Erfahrunge. *Allg Ztschr Psychiat* 1925–26;**83**:92–113.
9. Berrios GE. *The History of Mental Symptoms: descriptive psychopathology since the nineteenth century*, p.229. Cambridge: Cambridge University Press, 1996.
10. American Psychiatric Association. *Diagnostic and Statistical Manual of Mental Disorders*, pp.33–4. Washington, DC: American Psychiatric Association, 1952.
11. Healy D. *The Antidepressant Era*, p. 252. Cambridge, MA: Harvard University Press, 1997.
12. Ban T. From DSM-III to DSM-IV: progress or standstill? In: Franzck E, Ungvari GS, Rüther E, Beckman H (eds). *Progress in Differentiated Psychopathology*. Wuerzburg, Germany: International Werniche-Kleist-Leonhard Society, 2000: 1–11.
13. Olfson M, Marcus SC, Pincus HA. Trends in office-based psychiatric practice. *Am J Psychiatry* 1999;**156**:451–7.
14. Healy D. The three faces of the antidepressants: a critical commentary on the clinical-economic context of diagnosis. *J Nerv Ment Dis* 1999;**187**:174–80.
15. Knutson B, Wolkowitz OM, Cole SW *et al*. Selective alteration of personality and social behavior by serotonergic intervention. *Am J Psychiatry* 1998;**155**:373–9.
16. Shorter E. *A History of Psychiatry from the Era of the Asylum to the Age of Prozac*. New York: John Wiley, 1997.

Global burden of depressive disorders and future projections

T BEDIRHAN ÜSTÜN and SOMNATH CHATTERJI

The current magnitude of the problem

Depression is perhaps the most common form of mental disorder in the community and it is likely to increase its burden further in the forthcoming years.[1] Like hypertension, depressive illness can be seen as a deviation from the steady state of the body where brain functions (i.e. affect, cognition and motor functions) operate poorly. Depressive illness may therefore be seen as a 'brain disease' where mood regulation is locked in low mood and external stimuli are responded to by a response that is characterised by psychomotor retardation. There is overwhelming evidence at present that depression is indeed a disorder of the brain. A great deal of progress has been made in understanding its pathophysiological, molecular and genetic basis. Depression is now clearly recognised as an illness that goes with changes that occur in the serotonergic and other monoamine neurotransmitter systems in the brain that involves various cortical and subcortical structures. A genetic diathesis perhaps predisposes individuals to this condition and the full-blown disorder occurs in the context of life stressors.[2-9] Although it is not regarded as an officially recognised illness, some authors propose the existence of 'minor' or 'subthreshold' forms as well, which could be considered seriously both as a target for preventive intervention and for treatment[10] because they cause significant disability and dysfunctioning.

Though estimates of the prevalence and incidence of this condition vary depending on the definition and case finding methods, it is generally agreed that lifetime prevalences are between 2–15% for major depressive disorder.[11-17] More than three-quarters of these subjects report recurrent episodes over the life time with a risk of recurrence increasing with every successive episode. Each episode of depression lasts an average of six months with a small proportion of subjects having episodes of a long duration that can last up to several years. However, subjects continue to improve over the course of several years especially with adequate and rational treatment. Hence depressive disorders tend to be recurrent long-term illnesses and require both early identification and prompt and adequate treatment to avoid chronicity.[18-26]

Depressive disorders cause significant disability, i.e. they limit the activities and productivity of the persons. Disability associated with depression is greater than that reported for other chronic physical conditions such as hypertension, diabetes, arthritis and back pain. These results have been found in several studies in the United States[27, 28] as well as internationally in the WHO Psychological Problems in General Health Care (PPGHC) study.[29] Depression is also associated with a significant impact on the family, leading to a substantial carer burden.[30, 31]

Epidemiological issues

Regarding the incidence of depressive disorders, data are less often available and more likely to be unreliable given the nature of most epidemiological study methods. An incidence study conducted in Canada, in which 3956 community residents were interviewed using the Diagnostic Interview Schedule (DIS), and a sample of 1964 subjects were re-interviewed with the DIS an average of 2.8 years later, produced incidence rates that were surprisingly large, raising questions about the reliability of DIS data. There were 138 'incident' cases of major depression, giving an annual incidence rate for both sexes of 27.9 (per 1000). However, based on re-interview data, 106 (80%) of the incident cases reported an age of onset prior to the initial interview. These findings appear to be the result of a difference between the DIS definition of age of onset and the one used in this study. The large number of incident cases is probably due, at least in part, to incomplete recall of lifetime depressive symptoms.[32] Data from the NEMESIS study in the Netherlands suggest an incidence rate of 2.72 per 100 person-years at risk.[33] There is thus a great need to clearly estimate true incidence rates for population samples through longitudinal follow up studies in order to make reasonable predictions about future trends in the epidemiological scenario for depression.

In order to make reasonable future projections, we also need to know the secular and cohort trends in the occurrence of depressive disorders. However, these data are controversial.[34, 35, 36] The National Comorbidity Survey (NCS) data show that most cases of lifetime major depressive disorder (MDD) are secondary, i.e. they occur in people with a prior history of another DSM-III-R disorder. Secondary MDD is more persistent and severe than pure or primary MDD. This has special public health significance because it would suggest that though lifetime prevalence of secondary MDD has increased in recent cohorts, the prevalence of pure and primary depression has remained unchanged.[37] Elevated rates of MDD have also been shown to occur among those with co-morbid drug and alcohol abuse in both the family and community samples. However, the temporal increases in rates of MDD also occur in those with no such co-morbidity. Specifically, there are effects of age and gender. In addition, there is a period effect in family studies and a birth cohort effect in community samples. The recent increases in depression cannot be accounted for solely by concurrent increases in co-morbid drug and alcohol abuse. Temporal (period and cohort) effects on rates of depression do occur in addition to the contribution of co-morbid drug and alcohol abuse or dependence.[38]

Analysis of the Epidemiological Catchment Area (ECA) study in the United States suggests a sharp increase in rates of major depression among both men and women in the birth cohort born during the years 1935–45. The rates among females, however, seem to have stabilised in the generations born since 1945, while the rates in males have continued to rise sharply among the cohorts born in the following decade, after which, in 1955, they also levelled off. In contrast, the rates associated with period of onset of major depression continued to increase between the years 1960–80 among both men and women of all ages studied.[39] These findings are of particular interest given the persistent concentration of depression in women and in biologically related members of families of affected individuals.

However, other large-scale international studies suggest that apparent prevalence increases are non-specific.[40] Reporting patterns suggest significant undercounting of past depressive episodes. Respondents of all ages typically reported first onset of depression in the last five years. Reported lifetime prevalence was only 2.02 times current prevalence. These findings suggest that depression risk is not rapidly increasing and that true lifetime prevalence is probably much higher than estimated by cross-sectional surveys.

Methodological factors may largely influence the change in the prevalence of depression that has been reported with time. A simulation study to examine the magnitude of annual rates of forgetting that could produce the secular trends reported for MDD shows that small, but constant, annual rates produce striking 'cohort effect-like' curves. The rates needed to reconstruct the reported effect are compatible with published values for test–retest studies of lifetime recall of MDD.[41] This stresses the possible limitations of using cross-sectional studies to investigate secular trends.

Recent reanalysis of data from several studies suggests that when other risk factors are statistically controlled, there is a decrease in anxiety, depression and distress across age groups. This decrease cannot be accounted for by exclusion of elderly people in institutional care from epidemiological surveys or by selective mortality of people with anxiety or depression. There is, therefore, some evidence that aging is indeed associated with an intrinsic reduction in susceptibility to depression.[42] This is particularly important to consider given the aging of populations and its implications for the projection of future scenarios. Longitudinal studies covering the adult life span are needed to distinguish aging from cohort effects. More attention needs to be paid to understanding the mechanism behind any aging-related reduction in risk for anxiety and depression with age. Factors that have been speculated to be implicated are decreased emotional responsiveness with age, increased emotional control and psychological immunisation to stressful experiences.

Depression has also been shown to be highly co-morbid with other psychological and physical health conditions. Data from the NCS suggest that 58% of all subjects with a diagnosis of major depression also have a co-morbid psychiatric condition.[37] This has major implications for the estimate of burden of depression: depending on whether the co-morbidity is causal (as in the case of suicide and depression), non-causal (as in the case of diabetes and depression) or independent (as in the case of asthma and depression), the disability experienced may be additive, multiplicative or exponential. These relationships need to be examined carefully in large cohorts of depressive subjects that have been assessed for other chronic health conditions.

Depression also increases the risks for mortality from other health conditions. Recent analysis of the National Health Interview Survey (NHIS) in the United States shows that major depression increases the risk of all-cause mortality particularly among men (hazard rate ratio 3.1 for men and 1.7 for women) after adjusting for potential confounders such as age, marital status, education and body mass index).[43] Similar studies in The Netherlands also show that after adjusting for socio-demographic variables, health status and health behaviours such as smoking and physical inactivity, major depression was associated with a 1.83-fold higher mortality risk for older men and women.[44] This implies that the relative risk of dying because of depression is increased significantly further adding to the years of life lost due to this condition.

Further, several studies have pointed out that depression is under-recognised and undertreated perhaps consequent to lack of recognition by the physician and patient alike and due to characteristics of the health system in spite of effective treatments being available and relatively easy to use. This of course leads to further increase in disability and burden.[45]

The global burden of depressive disorders

The Global Burden of Disease (GBD) study was conducted by WHO and the World Bank to provide a set of summary health measures that would be comprehensive and provide information on disease and injury, including *non-fatal health outcomes*, to inform global priority setting for health research and to inform international health policy and planning. In order to ensure that these epidemiological assessments were unbiased and to uncouple them from advocacy, the GBD study developed internally consistent estimates of incidence, prevalence, duration and case fatality for 107 conditions and their 483 disabling consequences. These estimates of burden could also be used in cost-effectiveness analysis and to assess the attributable fraction of burden that is caused by risk factors.[46]

One of the major results of this exercise, once health estimates went beyond mortality to include morbidity (disability), was that conditions such as mental disorders, which disable but do not kill, were brought into sharp focus as a major cause of burden worldwide. Since traditional public health measures focused only on mortality, they never ranked mental disorders amongst the 'top ten' priority list. However, once 'disability' was entered into the equation, as is the case with the Disability Adjusted Life Year (DALY), mental disorders joined the rank of cardiovascular and respiratory diseases and in fact surpassed all malignancies combined, or HIV. The DALY methodology provides a way to link information on disease occurrences to information on short- and long-term outcomes including disabilities and restrictions in participation in usual life situations. WHO has over the years refined this framework for assessing the outcomes associated with health.[47]

DALYs are a common metric for fatal and non-fatal health outcomes and are based on years of life lost because of premature death (YLL) and years of life lived with disability (YLD). Thus

DALYs = YLL + YLD

and

Burden = Mortality + Disability.

Therefore, a DALY is one lost year of healthy life. The disability component is weighted according to the severity of the disability. For example, in the original GBD study, disability caused by major depression was weighted as being equivalent to blindness or paraplegia, whereas active psychosis, as seen in schizophrenia, was weighted somewhere between paraplegia and quadriplegia. Taking YLDs alone into account, depressive disorders, taken as a single diagnostic category, were the leading cause of disability worldwide.

Projections of burden of depressive disorders

The GBD study developed three alternative plausible projections of future mortality and disability, taking into account factors such as socio-economic development, educational attainment of the population and technological developments. Baseline, optimistic and pessimistic projections took such independent variables that are likely to influence mortality and disability in a major way into account for different age and sex groups, causes and regions. The findings suggest that the health trends in the next 20 years will be determined mainly by the aging of the world's population, the decline in age-specific mortality rates from communicable, maternal and nutritional disorders, the spread of HIV, and the increase in tobacco-related mortality and disability.[48] Significantly, it was predicted from the baseline model that in 2020, unipolar major depression will rank second after ischaemic heart disease in leading causes of DALYs, surpassing road-traffic accidents, cerebrovascular disease, chronic obstructive pulmonary disease, lower respiratory infections, tuberculosis, war injuries, diarrhoeal diseases and HIV, and increasing its share of DALYs due to all causes by more than 50%.[49]

Owing to changes in demography, epidemiological transitions,[50, 51, 52] and trends that can be reasonably estimated in various social factors such as family structures (breakdown of joint family and support structures into smaller units), urbanisation (a move from rural to urban areas of large population groups or changes in rural structures that will lead to a more urban structure of organisation), migration and mobility (related to factors such as socio-economic incentives, strife and conflict), and alcohol and drug use (that has been on the rise especially in youth and women), the risks for mental disorders will certainly increase. Coupled with these factors, an increase in population size, a longer life expectancy, possible increases in the rates of depression (as mentioned above under possible secular trends and cohort effects) and a relative decrease in other communicable disorders will result in depressive disorders being the leading cause of disability and overall burden worldwide. Data from 1990 show that, even among the poorest 20% of the global population, neuropsychiatric disorders (of which depression forms the major component) contributed to more DALYs lost than maternal conditions, tuberculosis, malaria, HIV, ischaemic heart disease or diabetes.[53] The results of the GBD study have shown variations by country and region, but the patterns and trends are very similar the world over. The findings call for continuing debate and further scientific studies to confirm and refine them. The GBD study has had certain limitations that need to be highlighted in order to appreciate its full impact.

Limitations of the GBD study

Data needs and methodology

The GBD study used basic regression equations to derive and evaluate the predictions. Measures of disease epidemiology (such as incidence, duration and course over time in terms of remission and severity) formed the basic parameters for these predictions. This methodology can be advanced by employing econometric methods that examine the link between health outcomes (such as disability), on the one hand, and determinants of health (such as environmental and behavioural risk factors, and socio-economic determinants) on the other. Also one can apply models derived from specific disease epidemics that have occurred in real populations (e.g. as demonstrated in the case of HIV).[54] The intent of all these methods is to generate estimates of mortality and disability in the world that are internally consistent.

However, the data used as input for the original GBD study to calculate the burden due to depressive disorders remain debatable: *episode incidence* was modelled as 0.29% for women and 0.16% for men; *average age at onset* was taken as 37.1 years and the *average episode duration* was considered to be six months.[55] Treatment rates for depressive disorders were counted as about 5% in subSaharan Africa and 35% in established market economies. These incidence and prevalence estimates are very low in comparison with the recent findings from epidemiological studies cited above. The annual prevalence of unipolar depression was 12.9% for women in the National Comorbidity Survey[10] as opposed to the 1.7% prevalence estimate used in the GBD calculations. Depression is now known to occur in younger age groups, often between 20 and 25 years, as compared to the estimate of 37.1.[56] This in fact means that the degree of burden estimated from the GBD results are *underestimates* for depressive disorders. The DISMOD computer program that was used to create internally consistent estimates of epidemiological parameters assumes a linear relation between incidence, duration and prevalence contributing to the discrepancy as well. In future iterations of the GBD study, more complex relations will be programmed. Data from empirical studies will be utilised to examine and model these relationships. Reliable and valid estimates of two-week prevalence rates of major depressive episodes, as well as the true incidence rates for this condition, through longitudinal studies that do not rely heavily on past recall, will provide valuable inputs into such a model.

The conceptualisation of depression

In the GBD study unipolar depression was modelled as an episodic illness. Current concepts of this disorder suggest that depression is better understood as a chronic relapsing medical illness. Data from both the NCS and ECA studies suggest that there is a small subgroup of major depressives who have a long-standing non-remitting illness (distinct from dysthymia). How these subjects should be accounted for in future models of burden is a challenge as they would greatly change the remission rates and incidence estimates – important parameters in the GBD model.

Another important consideration would be the continuum versus dichotomous debate in classifying depression. In other words, studies are needed to resolve questions surrounding whether depression is a single disorder that ranges from mild to moderate to severe (from minor to major), or whether major depression is a distinct entity that can then be graded into mild, moderate and severe (an approach taken by the International Classification of Diseases, ICD 10-DCR, for example.[57] This would then call for reliable estimates of incidence and prevalence by severity – considered a tall order by some.

Moreover, the GBD study considered depression only as an adult disease. There is overwhelming evidence at present that depression occurs with considerable frequency in childhood and adolescence; it can be reliably identified and is associated with increased disability, co-morbidity and poorer outcomes.[58] It is noteworthy too that life years lost because of suicide are not included in the depression burden to avoid double counting.

Use of a unitary disability weight

The disability weight for depressive disorder was taken as 0.6 for untreated cases and 0.3 for treated cases, irrespective of severity of depression (mild, moderate or severe) or age and world region in the original GBD study. Disability is a personal and social experience that is context sensitive and the weight needs to take this into account. Valuation exercises that use preference measures need to go beyond taking the perspective of healthcare professionals and their social preference to involving multiple perspectives of consumers, care providers, policymakers and other involved stakeholders. Models that estimate a strength of preference function, derived from actually measured disability as well as different forms of valuation exercises, need to be developed.

It is evident that various severity levels of illness are associated with different degrees of disability. Recent data from the Dutch burden of disease study show that the disability associated with mild, moderate and severe depression were accorded disability weights of 0.14, 0.35 and 0.76 respectively.[59] Outcomes of treatment vary by age or social circumstances. While it is possible to build more detailed models, using techniques such as Markov chain analysis for example, including these variables, the availability of data and the need to have a common framework across all disorders worldwide did not allow such detailed estimates.

Co-morbidity

The inclusion of co-morbidity in the GBD study has been limited. With few exceptions, i.e. Down syndrome with mental retardation and mental retardation with cerebral palsy, there is no explicit recognition of the impact of co-morbidity on disability in the GBD study. Given the high rates of co-morbidity of depressive disorders with other mental disorders and substance use disorders, as well as physical disorders, it is important to factor these phenomena in the calculation of GBD study. Empirical studies are required to estimate the extent of co-morbidity of depression with other psychiatric and physical health conditions, as well as to measure the experienced disability in such subjects, to understand the nature of the relationship with regard to calculation of YLDs.

Disregarding changes in disease trends

As mentioned, cohort effects and secular trends have been ignored in the GBD study. Future estimates will require valid estimates of these trends in order to model future scenarios of this condition accurately.

Overall, one cannot help reiterate that taking all the above factors into account, the GBD estimates were conservative, rather than overestimates, for depressive disorders.

Action for the future

The GBD study has brought to the fore a common framework for the comparison of mental with physical disorders. This has shown the relative importance of depressive disorders. It is time now to see how the findings can be applied to policymaking, planning and programme implementation. By improving the input variables of key importance, identifying key points of care provision and key strategies, we can certainly frame future scenarios by scanning for relevant emerging trends and develop policy options. Visioning the most likely future and alternative likely futures will allow us to evaluate the feasibility and desirability of an optimal path to a desired future.

How can we use this information for the management of health policy? How do we cope with the existing burden of depression? How do we decrease the future burden of depressive disorders? How can one incorporate care for depression within a comprehensive healthcare package? All these questions become all the more relevant when we realise that resources are limited: most countries in the world have less than US$ 20 per capita for their healthcare.

The evidence that depression must be one of the most important targets for the twenty-first century is overwhelming. Finding effective solutions to this major public health problem is necessary. Thinking about the future calls for profound reflection on policies and allocation of resources. Government agencies, care providers, consumers, industry and researchers should get together to find effective and sustainable ways to combat the increasing burden of depression.

The epidemiological parameters in projecting depression, such as population dynamics, age of onset, prevalence and risk factors may all be debated. However, under the most conservative estimates we still have the most alarming projection that the burden of depressive disorders will increase by at least 50% by 2020.

Given the gap between treatment efficacy (i.e. success in clinical research trials) and effectiveness (i.e. success in real-world settings) today, a programme of action for prevention and strategies of generalising effective treatment modalities are the need of the hour.[60] Current trends indicate that the treatment of depressive disorder must move to primary care. Evidence-based guidelines will increasingly be used in larger scales to inform care and policy. Relapses and chronicity of depressive disorders can be prevented with early identification and effective and rational treatment. The labour sector has already taken on workplace programmes geared towards preventing productivity loss and improving overall quality of life. Involvement of consumers and the awareness of self-help methods are growing.

We must think of innovative ways to deal with this problem. An important strategy is to strengthen the capacity of health systems to identify and manage depression, especially in developing countries where highly specialised human resources may not be available or even necessary. The technology to train primary healthcare professionals in the identification and management of depression is available. Guidelines for referral are available. Implementation of this technology, with regular monitoring mechanisms to demonstrate feasibility and effectiveness at national and international scales that go beyond small-scale experimentation, is urgently needed. There is a growing need to identify effective treatments and evaluate them within the framework of cost-effectiveness analysis (CEA), such that the treatment of depression can be evaluated against other interventions in terms of cost per DALY averted (see Figure 1).

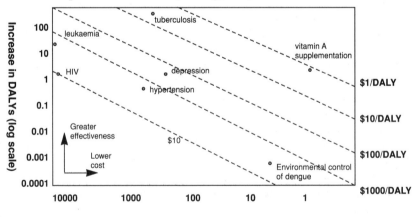

Figure 1 Comparative cost-effectiveness of various health interventions

To combat the burden of depressive disorders we must research the efficacy, effectiveness, cost-effectiveness and generalisability of both pharmacological and psycho-social interventions in different international and cross-cultural settings. We need to translate the findings from basic science into treatment and prevention interventions. Finally, we must investigate how these might best be implemented in the real world. The changing healthcare scene, with growing evidence-based medicine and policy, advancing information technology and developments in neuroscience and genetic research, may assist us in dealing with this burden. It is of interest to note that one of the four strongest predictors of risk of major depression in a co-twin, in a large twin study, was the degree of impairment caused by the disorder.[61] Most importantly, increased public awareness and consumer involvement will enable better dissemination and quality assurance for a generalisable and sustainable management strategy.

Acknowledgement

This paper is produced in the framework of WHO/NIH Joint Project on Assessment and Classification of Disability (UO1-MH 35883).

References

1. Üstün TB. The Worldwide Burden of Depression in the 21st Century. In: Weissman MM, ed. *Mental Health in the 21st Century*. Washington DC: American Psychiatric Press, 2000.
2. Andreasen NC. Linking mind and brain in the study of mental illnesses: a project for a scientific psychopathology. *Science* 1997;**275**:1586–93.
3. Leuchter AF, Cook IA, Uijtdehaage SH *et al*. Brain structure and function and the outcomes of treatment for depression. *J Clin Psychiatry* 1997;**58** (Suppl 16):22–31.
4. Risch SC. Recent advances in depression research: from stress to molecular biology and brain imaging. *J Clin Psychiatry* 1997;**58** (Suppl 5):3–6.
5. Duman RS, Heninger GR, Nestler EJ. A molecular and cellular theory of depression. *Arch Gen Psychiatry* 1997;**54**:597–606.
6. Kendler KS. Anna-Monika-Prize Paper. Major depression and the environment: a psychiatric genetic perspective. *Pharmacopsychiatry* 1998;**31**:5–9.
7. Mann JJ. Role of the serotonergic system in the pathogenesis of major depression and suicidal behavior. *Neuropsychopharmacology*. 1999;**21**:99S–105S.
8. Grasby PM. Imaging strategies in depression. *J Psychopharmacol* 1999;**13**:346–51.
9. Stahl SM. Blue genes and the monoamine hypothesis of depression. *J Clin Psychiatry* 2000;**61**:77–8.
10. Kessler RC, Walters EE. Epidemiology of DSM-III-R major depression and minor depression among adolescents and young adults in the National Comorbidity Survey. *Depress Anxiety* 1998;**7**:3–14.
11. Kessler RC, Zhao S, Blazer DG, Swartz M. Prevalence, correlates, and course of minor depression and major depression in the National Comorbidity Survey. *J Affect Disord* 1997;**45**:19–30.
12. Angst J. Epidemiology of depression. *Psychopharmacology* (*Berlin*) 1992;**106**:S71–S74.
13. Wittchen HU, Knauper B, Kessler RC. Lifetime risk of depression. *Br J Psychiatry* (Suppl.) 1994;16–22.
14. Eaton WW, Anthony JC, Gallo J *et al*. Natural history of Diagnostic Interview Schedule/DSM-IV major depression. The Baltimore Epidemiologic Catchment Area follow-up. *Arch Gen Psychiatry* 1997;**54**:993–9.

15. Szadoczky E, Papp Z, Vitrai J *et al.* The prevalence of major depressive and bipolar disorders in Hungary. Results from a national epidemiologic survey. *J Affect Disord.* 1998;**50**:153–62.
16. Takeuchi DT, Chung RC, Lin KM *et al.* Lifetime and twelve-month prevalence rates of major depressive episodes and dysthymia among Chinese Americans in Los Angeles. *Am J Psychiatry* 1998;**155**:1407–14.
17. Murphy JM, Laird NM, Monson RR *et al.* A 40-year perspective on the prevalence of depression: the Stirling County Study. *Arch Gen Psychiatry* 2000;**57**:209–15.
18. Coryell W, Endicott J, Keller MB. Predictors of relapse into major depressive disorder in a nonclinical population. *Am J Psychiatry* 1991;**148**:1353–8.
19. Coryell W, Akiskal HS, Leon AC *et al.* The time course of nonchronic major depressive disorder. Uniformity across episodes and samples. National Institute of Mental Health Collaborative Program on the Psychobiology of Depression – Clinical Studies. *Arch Gen Psychiatry* 1994;**51**:405–10.
20. Mueller TI, Keller MB, Leon AC *et al.* Recovery after 5 years of unremitting major depressive disorder. *Arch Gen Psychiatry* 1996;**53**:794–9.
21. Mueller TI, Leon AC. Recovery, chronicity, and levels of psychopathology in major depression. *Psychiatr Clin North America* 1996;**19**:85–102.
22. Solomon DA, Keller MB, Leon AC *et al.* Recovery from major depression. A 10-year prospective follow-up across multiple episodes. *Arch Gen Psychiatry* 1997;**54**:1001–6.
23. Judd LL, Akiskal HS, Maser JD *et al.* Major depressive disorder: a prospective study of residual subthreshold depressive symptoms as predictor of rapid relapse. *J Affect Disord* 1998;**50**:97–108.
24. Montgomery SA, Kasper S. Depression: a long-term illness and its treatment. *Int Clin Psychopharmacol* 1998;**13** (Suppl 6):S23–S6.
25. Mueller TI, Leon AC, Keller MB, *et al.* Recurrence after recovery from major depressive disorder during 15 years of observational follow-up. *Am J Psychiatry* 1999;**156**:1000–6.
26. Solomon DA, Keller MB, Leon AC *et al.* Multiple recurrences of major depressive disorder. *Am J Psychiatry* 2000;**157**:229–33.
27. Wells K Stewart A, Hays RD *et al.* The functioning and well-being of depressed patients. Results from the Medical Outcomes Study. *JAMA* 1989;**262**:914–19.
28. Spitzer RL, Kroenke K, Linzer M *et al.* Health-related quality of life in primary care patients with mental disorders. Results from the PRIME-MD 1000 Study. *JAMA* 1995;**274**:1511–17.
29. Üstün TB, Sartorius N. *Mental Illness in General Health Care.* Chichester: John Wiley 1995.
30. Jacob M, Frank E, Kupfer DJ, Carpenter LL. Recurrent depression: an assessment of family burden and family attitudes. *J Clin Psychiatry* 1987;**48**:395–400.
31. Chisholm D, Kumar K, Sekar K *et al.* Integration of mental healthcare into primary care: a demonstration cost-outome study in India and Pakistan. *Br J Psychiatry* 2000 (in press).
32. Newman SC, Bland RC. Incidence of mental disorders in Edmonton: estimates of rates and methodological issues. *J Psychiatr Res* 1998;**32**:273–82.
33. Bijl RV, Ravelli A, van Zessen G. Prevalence of psychiatric disorder in the general population: results of The Netherlands Mental Health Survey and Incidence Study (NEMESIS). *Psychiatry Psychiatr Epidemiol* 1998;**33**:587–95.
34. Stassen HH, Ragaz M, Reich T. Age-of-onset or age-cohort changes in the lifetime occurrence of depression? *Psychiatr Genet* 1997;**7**:27–34.
35. Fombonne E. Increased rates of depression: update of epidemiological findings and analytical problems. *Acta Psychiatr Scand* 1994;**90**:145–56.
36. Simon GE, Von Korff M. Reevaluation of secular trends in depression rates. *Am J Epidemiol* 1992;**135**:1411–22.
37. Kessler RC, Nelson CB, McGonagle KA *et al.* Comorbidity of DSM-III-R major depressive disorder in the general population: results from the US National Comorbidity Survey. *Br J Psychiatry* (Suppl) 1996;**30**:17–30.
38. Klerman GL, Leon AC, Wickramaratne P *et al.* The role of drug and alcohol abuse in recent increases in depression in the US. *Psychol Med* 1996;**26**:343–51.
39. Wickramaratne PJ, Weissman MM, Leaf PJ, Holford TR. Age, period and cohort effects on the risk of major depression: results from five United States communities. *J Clin Epidemiol* 1989;**42**:333–43.

40. Simon GE, Von Korff M, Üstün TB *et al.* Is the lifetime risk of depression actually increasing? *J Clin Epidemiol* 1995;**48**:1109–18.
41. Giuffra LA, Risch N. Diminished recall and the cohort effect of major depression: a simulation study. *Psychol Med* 1994;**24**:375–83.
42. Jorm AF. Does old age reduce the risk of anxiety and depression? A review of epidemiological studies across the adult life span. *Psychol Med* 2000;**30**:11–22.
43. Zheng D, Macera CA, Croft JB *et al.* Major depression and all cause mortality among white adults in the United States. *Ann Epidemiol* 1997;**7**:213–18.
44. Pennix BWJH, Geerlings SW, Deeg DJH *et al.* Minor and major depression and the risk of death in older persons. *Arch Gen Psychiatry* 1999;**56**:889–95.
45. Davidson JRT, Meltzer-Brody SE. The underrecognition and undertreatment of depression: what is the breadth and depth of the problem? *J Clin Psychiatry* 1999; **60** (Suppl 7):4–9.
46. Murray CJL, Lopez AD, eds: *The Global Burden of Disease.* Cambridge, MA: Harvard University Press, 1996.
47. World Health Organization. *ICIDH-2: International Classification of Functioning and Disability. Beta-2 draft, Full Version.* Geneva: World Health Organization, 1999.
48. Murray CJL, Lopez AD. Alternative projections of mortality and disability by cause 1990–2020: Global Burden of Disease study. *Lancet* 1997;**349**:1498–1504.
49. World Health Organization. *The World Health Report 1999: making a difference.* Geneva: World Health Organization, 1999.
50. Kalache A. Demographic transition poses a challenge to societies worldwide. *Trop Med Int Health* 1997;**2**:925–6.
51. Manton KG, Stallard E, Corder L. Changes in the age dependence of mortality and disability: cohort and other determinants. *Demography* 1997;**34**:135–57.
52. Omran AR. The epidemiologic transition: a theory of the epidemiology of population change. *Milbank Memorial Fund Quarterly* 1971;**49**:509–38.
53. Gwatkin DR, Guillot M. *The Burden of Disease among the Global Poor. Current situation, future trends, and implications for strategy.* Washington, DC: The World Bank, 2000.
54. Salomon JA, Gakidou EE, Murray CJ. Methods for modeling the HIV/AIDS epidemic in sub-Saharan Africa. GPE Discussion Paper No. 3. Geneva: World Health Organization, 1999.
55. Murray CJL, Lopez AD. *Global Health Statistics: a compendium of incidence, prevalence and mortality estimates for over 200 conditions,* pp.601–6. Cambridge: Harvard School of Public Health, 1996.
56. Burke KC, Burke, JD Jr, Rae DS, Regier DA. Comparing age at onset of major depression and other psychiatric disorders by birth cohorts in five US community populations. *Arch Gen Psychiatry* 1991;**48**:789–95.
57. World Health Organization. *The ICD-10 Classification of Mental and Behavioural Disorders: diagnostic criteria for research.* Geneva: World Health Organization, 1993.
58. Costello EJ, Erkanli A, Federman E, Angold A. Development of psychiatric comorbidity with substance abuse in adolescents: effects of timing and sex. *J Clin Child Psychol.* 1999;**28**:298–311.
59. Stouthard M, Essink-Bot M, Bonsel G *et al. Disability Weights for Diseases in Netherlands.* Rotterdam: Department of Public Health, Erasmus University, 1997.
60. Üstün TB. Global burden of mental disorders. *Am J Public Health.* 1999;**89**:1315–18.
61. Kendler KS, Gardner CO, Prescott CA. Clinical characteristics of major depression that predict risk of depression in relatives. *Arch Gen Psychiatry* 1999;**56**:322–7.

Fifty years of depression

DAVID HEALY

Abstract/summary

Estimates of the prevalence of depressive disorders have mushroomed from 100 per million from the late 1950s to over 100 000 per million in the late 1990s. There is compelling evidence that the incidence of major melancholic and bipolar depressions has not changed between 1950 and 1990. The changes are in the realm of minor to moderate nervous disorders where what were formerly termed 'anxiety' or 'neurotic disorders' have been transformed into depressive disorders. The vast majority of these conditions are managed in primary care, where campaigns are run to improve rates at which primary care practitioners detect patients with depressive disorders and institute treatment. The aim of such campaigns is to reduce national suicide rates and the disability that stems from depression. Treatment with antidepressants, however, can in its own right be associated with considerable drug-induced disability, including suicide and suicidality. It is not clear that primary care practitioners have been properly trained for this task.

In the 1950s, the best estimates of the incidence of depressive disorders put the figure at no more than 100 people per million. Current prevalence figures run to 100 000 people per million for depressive disorders and even higher for depressive symptoms.[1] We live in an Age of Depression. Depression is touted as one of the most significant sources of disability within the health domain.[2] Detection and treatment of depressive conditions is advocated on the basis that this will lead to a reduction in national suicide rates. Has there been a real increase in the prevalence of

45

depression and will our current treatment arsenal permit us to make inroads on the level of depressive-related disability or lower national suicide rates?

The incidence of severe bipolar, psychotic and melancholic disorders has probably remained essentially the same over the course of the century.[3] The change between 1950 and now therefore lies in the area of detection. There was almost certainly a substantial volume of undetected severe depressive morbidity in the 1950s and earlier, and a proportion of these conditions are now detected, in part as a result of national campaigns in a number of countries to increase rates of detection. A considerable proportion, however, would appear to remain undetected, as studies of suicides indicate that a far smaller proportion are on antidepressant treatment at the time of death than would be expected.[4]

There are two further sources for increased rates of detection. When faced with the discovery of agents that might be of benefit for depressive disorders, pharmaceutical companies were initially reluctant to develop these agents as the market size appeared insufficient to guarantee a reasonable return.[3] During the decade after the emergence of the antidepressants, however, there was a slow increase in the rates of diagnosis of depression, reflecting perhaps the fact that the simple availability of these drugs facilitated an increase in rates of diagnosis.[5] In the mid-1970s, the first body aimed at enhancing rates of detection and treatment of depression, the Prevention and Treatment of Depression committee, was set up by Paul Kielholz, Norman Sartorius and others. This international committee and programme, supported by Ciba-Geigy, was a forerunner of the national programmes that came into being in the 1990s.

Up to the 1980s, the majority of primary care nervous conditions were seen by clinicians and sufferers alike as anxiety disorders, with speculation from philosophers through to the media on the reasons why the period was an Age of Anxiety. By the early 1980s, the benzodiazepines, which had been the leading treatments for this condition, were falling out of favour for a variety of reasons, among which were fears of dependence. At this point the selective serotonin-reuptake inhibitors (SSRIs) were developed, with options for development as anxiolytics or antidepressants. The climate dictated an option for depression.[6]

The origins of the SSRIs lay in observations by Kielholz and Carlsson of correspondences between different functional and biochemical effects among the then available tricyclic antidepressants (TCAs). This led to the synthesis and development of zimelidine and a subsequent series of SSRIs. This new group of drugs was not produced to be safer, side effect-free versions of the older TCAs. They were specifically produced to have different functional effects to the TCAs. Retrospectively, this action can be best characterised as a serenic effect. Consistent with this, the SSRIs have since been shown to be effective for obsessive–compulsive disorder, panic disorder, social phobia, post-traumatic stress disorder and other conditions where noradrenergic-selective TCAs are ineffective. Given the availability of effective treatments, the apparent incidence of some of these conditions has also increased a thousandfold.[7]

As with depression, this reflects a combination of the availability of agents to meet unmet needs and astute marketing. In the case of depression, the collapse of the anxiolytic market in the mid-to-late 1980s left the way open for the market development of depression. In Japan, problems with benzodiazepine dependence never emerged and the market for anxiolytics remains a much bigger one than that for depression, with the first SSRI (fluvoxamine) being made available there only in 1999.

Coincidentally, a number of national psychiatric and primary case associations instituted campaigns to defeat depression, based in great part on work from Sweden suggesting that enhanced rates of detection and effective treatment could lower suicide rates.[8] Earlier work by Guze and Robins[9] had suggested that affective disorders are associated with a 15% lifetime prevalence of suicide. This figure has been widely cited – out of context. The 15% figure was derived from studies of hospitalised depressions, many of them conducted before the advent of antidepressants. Until recently, we have lacked a figure for suicide rates for primary care depressions.

It must first be emphasised that the SSRIs were among the first psychotropic agents to be rationally developed and their emergence has significantly enhanced therapeutic capability. Second, the group of agents termed SSRIs differ in the range of their functional effects and side-effects. But against these two factors must be set the fact that these agents have been marketed as being particularly safe for primary care depression, owing to safety in overdose, and as freer of drug-induced disability than the older TCAs.

As regards suicide, there is no evidence that the mass detection of primary care 'depression' and the institution of unmonitored treatment has led to a lowering of suicide rates. In fact, a substantial case can be made that at least one SSRI, fluoxetine, can induce suicidality and violence.[10] Based on published figures for suicide rates on antidepressants in British primary care,[11] which give estimates of 187 per 100 000 patient years on fluoxetine compared with indications that the suicide rate for primary care depression should be around 30 per 100 000 patient years, along with data on suicide attempts on SSRIs [12,13], it can be estimated that of those started on fluoxetine, up to 1000 people per million more than the rate for untreated depression or depression treated with other agents, go on to commit suicide and up to 10 000 per million make suicide attempts.

It may in fact be all but impossible to lower primary care suicide rates. The hazards of the first few weeks of antidepressant treatment have led to physician guidelines in Germany, the Netherlands and a number of other countries, requiring prescribers to see patients within one or two weeks. Such standards do not exist in the United Kingdom or the United States.

Furthermore there have been no educational campaigns to warn prescribers of the risks of treatment.

Equally, while it is clear that effective antidepressant treatment may reduce the disability induced by severe mood disorders, it is far from clear that mass detection and treatment will not in fact increase disability. Antidepressant trials to date have demonstrated treatment effects rather than treatment efficacy, effectiveness or efficiency. And where treatment effects have been demonstrated, the demonstrations depend on the use of physician-based rating scales. Quality of life scales have also been extensively employed in trials of mild-to-moderate depression. These give patient-based assessments of outcome. The results, however, have remained largely unpublished, suggesting that treatment may not be associated with the clear cut resolution of disability suggested by the marketing of antidepressants.[7]

References

1. Kessler RC, McGonagle KA, Zhao S. Lifetime and 12-month prevalence of DSM-III-R psychiatric disorders in the United States: results from the National Co-morbidity study. *Arch Gen Psychiatry* 1994; **51**:8–19.
2. Murray CJL, Lopez AD, eds. *The Global Burden of Disease*. Cambridge, MA: Harvard University Press, 1996.
3. Healy D. *The Antidepressant Era*. Cambridge, MA: Harvard University Press, 1997.
4. Isacsson G, Holmgren P, Wasserman D, Bergman U. Use of antidepressants among people committing suicide in Sweden. *BMJ* 1994;**308**:506–509.
5. Hare EH. The changing content of psychiatric illness. *J Psychosom Res* 1974;**18**:283–9.
6. Healy D. The marketing of 5HT:anxiety or depression? *Br J Psychiatry* 1991;**158**:737–42.
7. Healy D. The three faces of the antidepressants: a critical commentary on the clinical–economic context of diagnosis. *J Nerv Ment Dis* 1999;**187**:174–80.
8. Rutz W, von Knorring L, Pihlgren H *et al.* An educational project on depression and its consequences: is frequency of major depression among Swedish men underrated resulting in high suicidality? *Primary Care Psychiatry* 1995;**1**:59–63.
9. Guze SB, Robins E. Suicide and primary affective disorders. *Br J Psychiatry* 1970;**117**:437–8.
10. Healy D, Langmaak C, Savage M. Suicide in the course of the treatment of depression. *J Psychopharmacol* 1999;**13**:94–9.
11. Jick SS, Dean AD, Jick H. Antidepressants and suicide. *BMJ* 1995;**310**:215–8.
12. Healy, D. A failure to warn. *Int J Risk Safety Med* 1999;**12**:151–6.
13. Kasper S. The place of milnacipran in the treatment of depression. *Hum Psychopharmacol* 1997;**12**(Suppl 3):S135–S141.

Depression and the elderly

DAVID AMES

Who are the elderly?

Whether old age is defined chronologically or physiologically, the numbers of older people on our planet are at unprecedented levels and will grow more rapidly than other age cohorts in the twenty-first century.[1] From 550 million in 1996, the world's population aged above 60 years is expected to reach 1.2 billion by 2025.[1] Most developed countries already have 15–22% of their citizens in this age group.[1] The fastest growth in aged populations is occurring in the developing world. Indonesia's elderly will increase by over 400% between 1990 and 2025 and those aged above 60 years in China by more than 200% in the same period.[2] Within this burgeoning cohort of older people, the most rapid growth will occur in the numbers of very old people (over 80 years) who are at high risk of age-related disease and disability.[2] Managing the age-related health needs of an unprecedentedly large and rapidly growing aged population will be one of the key public health challenges of the next fifty years.

Is late life depression any different from depression at earlier ages?

Some authors have reported less subjective lowering of mood, fewer suicidal thoughts, more hypochondriasis, somatic complaints, weight loss and constipation, as well as more frequent subjective and objective cognitive difficulty among older people with depression when compared with younger depressed individuals.[3] Most of these studies examined hospital inpatients and may have been biased by different admission thresholds for patients of

49

different ages.[3] A community-based epidemiological study of 2725 people aged 18–79 years in Canberra, Australia, found symptoms of depression to decline with age in both men and women. Complaints of early waking, poor sleep, feeling slowed up, hopeless or miserable, having suicidal thoughts and losing interest in things were more likely to be endorsed by older people, while weight loss was a less common complaint for the old than the young.[4] Despite this, the overall consensus of a prolonged and continuing debate is that depression at all ages has similar core features.[3] However, the elderly are more likely than the young to have co-morbid dementia or physical ill health, or to have been recently bereaved, and modern diagnostic criteria[5,6] proscribe the allocation of a primary depressive diagnosis in some of these circumstances. Thus some elderly people with depressive syndromes may be classified as having an organic mood disorder, dementia with depressed mood or a normal bereavement reaction rather than a primary depressive disorder.

Epidemiology

Studies that assess rates of depressive disorders using standardised international criteria such as DSM-IV major depressive disorder[5] and ICD-10 depressive disorder[6] tend to find rates of depression between 0.5 and 3% of the community dwelling elderly.[3,7] These rates are somewhat lower than those found among younger age cohorts.[3,7] Broader criteria, which include those with significant depressive symptoms that interfere with daily functioning and may be present in the context of conditions that DSM-IV and ICD-10 specifically exclude from classification as primary depressive disorder, tend to find rates in the 6% to 20% range.[3,7–9] These milder depressions have been defined as justifying some sort of treatment intervention.[3,9–11] As with other age groups women are more often affected than men, in the approximate ratio 7: 3.[3,7] Physical ill health (especially chronic pain, urinary incontinence and conditions producing chronic activity limitation), stressful life events and poor social support are associated with depressive disorders in late life.[3,7,8] Studies using similar methodology have found more depression among old people in North America and northern Europe than in southern Europe or South East Asia.[3,9] All studies that assess institutional populations find depression (however defined) to be far more common in those who dwell in residential and nursing homes.[10] Depression is also more frequent among old people in general hospital wards than it is in those living at home.[11]

Aetiology

Genetic susceptibility to depressive disorder appears to diminish with age.[7] Age-associated alterations in cortisol levels and thyroid functioning parallel neuroendocrine abnormalities found in some depressed individuals.[7,12]

Structural brain changes, especially deep white matter lesions seen on magnetic resonance imaging (MRI), are more common in elderly depressed patients than in age-matched controls and appear to be a specific risk factor for the onset of a first ever depressive disorder in old age.[7,13] These lesions may reflect the presence of subtle cerebrovascular disease.[13] The association of a range of physical conditions and social situations with depression in late life was noted above. One might conjecture that societal attitudes to aging in increasingly narcissistic developed societies may foster a climate in which the experience of aging itself is likely to be viewed negatively by those growing older and thus could act as a potential risk factor for the development of a mood disorder.[14]

Detection and assessment

Perhaps the majority of elderly people with a depressive syndrome may not declare their symptoms spontaneously to their general practitioner and studies in primary care tend to suggest that a substantial proportion of depressive morbidity in older people is either undetected or undertreated.[10,15–17] A high index of suspicion and a willingness to ask about depressive symptoms are prerequisites for effective detection, and targeted awareness programmes may improve detection and treatment rates.[17] Enquiry about suicidal feelings and an attempt to detect common co-morbid or confounding disorders such as dementia form essential components of the assessment process. Informant histories are vital in psychiatric assessment at all ages but are especially useful in older patients whose self-reported histories may be unduly coloured by depressive cognitions or clouded by co-morbid cognitive decline.[7]

Management

Management of late life depression should utilise some combination of physical, psychological and social interventions.[3,18] Detection and optimal treatment of co-morbid physical complaints is an important but sometimes neglected component of physical care.[7,10] The evidence base from randomised controlled trials (RCTs) of antidepressant therapy for the depressed elderly is flawed by a reliance on highly selected patient samples in which those in institutions and patients with co-morbid physical illness or dementia are underrepresented.[3,18] Available data from over 70 RCTs suggest that antidepressants are efficacious in 50–60% of cases compared to a recovery rate of around 30% on placebo.[3] Newer antidepressants such as selective serotonin-reuptake inhibitors appear to be better tolerated by the old than the more established tricyclic drugs but there is a need for additional research, especially on the efficacy and tolerability of antidepressants in those with depression and dementia or serious physical illness.[3] Because of high relapse rates in elderly people who recover from depression,[3] maintenance therapy has been recommended for at least six months after an initial depressive episode and for much longer after subsequent depressions, though these recommendations are supported by a relatively slender evidence base.[7,19]

Available evidence suggests that electroconvulsive therapy is the most effective treatment for the severely depressed older patient, especially if delusions or hallucinations are present.[3,7] Initial suprathreshold unilateral application is recommended.[3] Again, the available RCTs are less than ideal and more research on this topic is required.[3]

Psychosocial interventions, especially cognitive behavioural therapy,[19] have been found efficacious in some RCTs but insufficient attention has been paid to the potentially confounding effects of physical ill health, extreme age and cognitive decline.[19]

Because much late life depression is multifactorial in origin, and because individual patients are likely to require management that is more specifically tailored to their individual requirements than the 'one size fits all' approach adopted in most pharmacological RCTs, multifaceted interventions in representative populations need thorough prospective evaluation. Such studies are extremely difficult to do, but two recent additions to the literature reveal that they are not impossible to plan and execute.[17,20] Receipt of an individual package of care formulated by a psychogeriatric team proved nine times more likely to be associated with recovery from depression than standard general practitioner care provided to a group of 69 depressed frail elderly receiving home care in south London.[20] This result did not seem to be due to simple prescribing of an antidepressant.[20] An elegant evaluation of a shared care intervention package that incorporated multidisciplinary collaboration, general practitioner training and resident education and activity programmes reported significantly more movement to less depressed levels than was seen in a control group among 220 depressed residents of a retirement complex in Sydney.[17]

Outcome including suicide

Studies of the long-term outcome of depression in the elderly have been bedevilled by poor methodology, small sample sizes and an overemphasis on inpatient samples. All such prognostic studies have been undertaken in developed countries and data from the developing world are scant.[3]

Where late life depression has received inpatient treatment from psychiatrists, follow-up studies of one to two years' duration find around 22% of patients remain continuously depressed for up to two years, approximately 44% recover and remain well, 16% undergo at least one depressive relapse and 23% have other outcomes such as death or dementia.[21] Among cohorts with over two years of follow up, 14% have continuous unremitting depression, 27% maintain long-term remission after initial recovery, 33% have at least one relapse and 31% experience other outcomes.[21] Poor outcome associates inconsistently with physical illness severity, cognitive impairment and severity of depression.[21] The longer people have been ill before treatment the less likely they are to do well.[3] Severe deep white matter lesions found on MRI are associated with very poor long-term outcomes.[22] Severe intervening life events are associated with worse outcomes but other social variables have little apparent impact.[21] There is a dearth of studies examining the long-term outcome of late life depression in primary care, but a Dutch study using 14 general practitioners found that 21 of 39 depressed elderly patients had recovered after 18 months of standard care.

In five community studies, depressed elderly individuals were identified in epidemiological surveys and then reviewed at a later date. Where follow up was of two years or shorter duration, 27% were continuously depressed, 34% recovered from depression and 31% had other outcomes, which included death, dementia, depressive relapse after initial recovery or development of a new psychiatric disorder.[21] Longer follow ups found 27% to have continuous depression, 19% to be free of depression and 44% had other outcomes.[21] Rates of antidepressant prescribing in these studies were low (4–33%) and the presence of physical illness made poor outcomes more likely.[21]

In most countries with available data, males aged over 75 are at higher risk of suicide than other population groups.[22] Up to 90% of these individuals are suffering from a depressive disorder and the majority consult a health professional within a few weeks of their death, raising the possibility that some of these suicides could be prevented.[3,7]

Conclusions

The rapid increase in numbers of older people worldwide indicates that late life depression will be a more prevalent disorder in the twenty-first century than it is now. Current best practice would advocate that healthcare professionals should evaluate older people for depressive symptoms, especially when they are in high-risk groups. Antidepressants are helpful for the more severe types of late life depression and emerging evidence on multifaceted interventions suggests that these show significant promise for milder depressions in primary care settings. High relapse rates after initial recovery and the alarming frequency with which elderly males end their own lives are urgent reminders of the need to improve our detection and long-term management of depressive disorders in the elderly. The possibility that some cases of late life depression may be linked to the presence of subtle cerebrovascular disease implies the possibility of improved prevention of such disorders in future.

References

1. World Health Organization. Ad hoc Committee on Health Research relating to Future Intervention Options. *Investing in Health Research and Development*. Geneva: World Health Organization, 1996.
2. US Census Bureau. *Global Aging into the 21st Century*. Washington, DC: National Institute on Aging, 1996.
3. Chiu E, Ames D, Draper B, Snowdon J. Depressive disorders in the elderly: a review. In: Maj M, Sartorius N, eds. *Depressive Disorders*, pp.313–63. Chichester: John Wiley, 1999.
4. Henderson AS, Jorm AF, Korten AE *et al* Symptoms of depression and anxiety during adult life: evidence for a decline in prevalence with age. *Psychol Med* 1998;**28**:1321–28.
5. American Psychiatric Association. *Diagnostic and Statistical Manual of Mental Disorders: DSM-IV*, 4th edn. Washington, DC: American Psychiatric Association, 1994.
6. World Health Organization. *The ICD-10 Classification of Mental and Behavioural Disorders: clinical descriptions and diagnostic guidelines*. Geneva: World Health Organization, 1992.
7. Baldwin R. Depressive illness. In: Jacoby R, Oppenheimer C, eds. *Psychiatry in the Elderly*, 2nd edn, pp. 536–73. Oxford: Oxford University Press, 1997.
8. Lepine JP, Bouchez S. Epidemiology of depression in the elderly. *Int Clin Psychopharmacol* 1998;**13**(Suppl 5):S7–S12.
9. Kua EH. A community study of mental disorders in elderly Singaporean Chinese using the GMS-AGECAT package. *Aust NZ J Psychiatry* 1992;**26**:502–6.
10. Ames D. Depression in nursing and residential homes. In: Chiu E, Ames D, eds. *Functional Psychiatric Disorders of the Elderly: symposium papers*, pp.142–6. New York: Cambridge University Press, 1994.
11. Ames D, Tuckwell V. Psychiatric disorders among elderly patients in a general hospital. *Med J Aust* 1994;**160**:671–5.
12. Philpot M. The biology of functional psychiatric disorders. In: Chiu E, Ames D, eds. *Functional Psychiatric Disorders of the Elderly: symposium papers*, pp.355–76. New York: Cambridge University Press, 1994.
13. O'Brien J, Ames D, Desmond P *et al*. A magnetic resonance imaging study of white matter lesions in depression and Alzheimer's disease. *Br J Psychiatry* 1996;**168**:477–85.
14. Ames D, Chiu E. Depression in the elderly. *Mental Health in Australia* 1994;**6**:12–17.
15. MacDonald AJ. Do general practitioners 'miss' depression in elderly patients? *Br Med J (Clin Res Ed)* 1986;**292**:1365–67.
16. Blanchard M, Mann AH. Depression in primary care settings. In: Chiu E, Ames D, eds. *Functional Psychiatric Disorders of the Elderly: symposium papers*, pp.163–76. New York: Cambridge University Press, 1994.
17. Llewellyn-Jones RH, Baikie KA, Smithers H *et al*. Multifaceted shared care intervention for late life depression in residential care: randomised controlled trial. *BMJ* 1999;**319**:676–82.
18. NIH Consensus Conference. Diagnosis and treatment of depression in late life. *JAMA* 1992;**268**:1018–24.
19. Koder D, Brodaty H, Anstey K. Cognitive therapy for depression in the elderly. *Int J Geriatr Psychiatry* 1996;**11**:97–107.
20. Banerjee S, Shamash K, Macdonald AJ, Mann AH. Randomised controlled trial of effect of intervention by psychogeriatric team on depression in frail elderly people at home. *BMJ* 1996;**313**:1058–61.
21. Cole MG, Bellavance F. The prognosis of depression in old age. *Am J Geriatr Psychiatry* 1997;**5**:4–14.
22. O'Brien J, Ames D, Chiu E *et al*. Severe deep white matter lesions and outcome in elderly patients with major depressive disorder: followup study. *BMJ* 1998;**317**:982–4.

Somatisation and depression

STEVEN REID and SIMON WESSELY

A man's body and his mind are exactly like a jerkin and a jerkin's lining:
rumple the one, you rumple the other.

The Life and Opinions of Tristram Shandy, Gentleman
Laurence Sterne

The management of somatisation is one of the most common problems encountered in medical practice, yet also presents one of the greatest challenges. Generally regarded as the expression of psychological distress through physical symptoms, somatisation is recognised as a universal phenomenon.[1-3] Its association with psychiatric illness, particularly depression, has been well documented[4-7] and we also know that lack of an effective intervention leads to a substantial number of unproductive consultations and investigations.[8-10] However, somatisation remains subject to a number of misconceptions, which as well as contributing to the undertreatment of affective disorders,[11] reinforce the belief that symptom complaints reflect either physical or psychological disorder and never a combination of the two.

Conceptual issues and terminology remain obstacles to progress in our understanding of somatisation. The term itself has been subject to multiple definitions with different meanings. Bridges and Goldberg[6] proposed the following operational definition, which has been used for many of the epidemiological studies in the area: (1) the patient must present with somatic manifestations of psychiatric illness, and not psychological symptoms; (2) the patient considers that their symptoms are caused by a physical problem; (3) they must report symptoms that justify a psychiatric diagnosis; and (4) treatment of the psychiatric disorder would result in the remission of the somatic symptoms. Others[12] have defined somatisation as the articulation of personal and social distress through physical symptoms – allowing for the absence of notable affective symptoms– or have placed an emphasis on the denial of psychological distress and the substitution of somatic symptoms. The psychiatric classification systems (ICD-10 and DSM-IV) have proven unhelpful, particularly in primary care, with their focus upon the chronic somatoform disorders such as hypochondriasis and somatisation disorder.[13] There is often a tacit assumption that the more common, acute somatisers represent early, less severe forms of the somatoform disorder but as yet there is little evidence to support this. What is clear is that the acute forms of somatisation are much more common and account for a substantial proportion of the undiagnosed psychiatric morbidity in primary care.[14]

The association of depression with physical symptoms is well established. As many as 80% of depressed or anxious primary care attenders initially present with exclusively somatic complaints.[6,7] Numerous studies[15-17] have found a high prevalence of depression in samples of patients presenting with unexplained physical symptoms and multiple symptoms are known to further increase the risk of psychiatric comorbidity.[18,19] Far too many studies to quote find that physical symptoms are an integral part of the experience of depression – it is easiest to say that we know of no study that reports anything different.

Figures vary according to definition but Bridges and Goldberg reported that somatisation had a prevalence of 19% amongst primary care attenders in Manchester.[6] Kirmayer and Robbins found a similar rate – 26.3%[20] in their US study. Somatising patients are typically regarded as young, female and less well educated. However, these findings are derived from studies of somatisation disorder,[21-23] a diagnosis rarely made outside of specialist settings (prevalence of 0.1–0.7%). Large-scale, epidemiological studies have not confirmed these findings. Piccinelli and Simon, as part of a World Health Organization study,[24] investigated somatic symptoms associated with emotional distress in 14 countries and found that once levels of emotional distress were controlled for, gender no longer had a significant effect. The perception that somatisation occurs more frequently in non-Western countries or the developing world has also persisted despite evidence to the contrary.[2,3] Higher rates of somatisation are found in studies of immigrant populations but after controlling for factors such as education and employment, most of the differences between immigrants as a group and the indigenous population disappear.[1] Variations in levels of somatisation across cultural groups have been found, although with no clear trend accounting for the difference, but Simon et al.[3] observed a tendency for somatic presentation to occur more frequently at centres offering walk-in care rather than a more personal form of care. This highlights the importance of the doctor–patient interaction to modes of presentation, and suggests a potential drawback to the new National Health Service (NHS) 'Walk In' centres that bypass the family doctor.

A number of interpretations have been put forward to explain why some patients present with somatic complaints in articulating their distress and others are more likely to report psychological symptoms. Goldberg and Bridges[14] view somatisation as a means of avoiding blame – preventing the sufferer from being perceived as mentally ill and allowing them to be relieved of responsibility for their predicament. Kirmayer and Young[1] have emphasised the role of somatisation in the communication of experience. Any explanation needs to take account of illness beliefs (both patient and doctor), an area often left unexplored in medical practice.

Genetics

In an adoption study Cloninger et al.[25] reported a familial association between somatisation, alcohol misuse and antisocial personality. More recently, a twin-family study[26] reported that somatisation was significantly influenced by genetic factors, with familial–environmental factors having little role. However, somatisation was measured by self-report on a five-item scale, which raises questions about the validity of the finding. At present, therefore, there are insufficient data upon which to draw any conclusions about the role of genetics in somatisation.

Pathophysiological mechanisms

The idea that medically unexplained somatic symptoms are 'all in the mind' is now outdated. There is evidence that in these patients physiological processes such as autonomic arousal, hyperventilation and smooth muscle contraction may give rise to increased bodily sensations.[27,28] These findings illustrate the need for an integrated approach to research and management of these disorders.

Early life experience

It has long been recognised that future illness behaviour is influenced by parental attitudes to childhood sickness.[29] A number of retrospective studies have indicated that children exposed to serious physical illness or persistent somatic complaints in family members are at greater risk of somatisation in later life.[30,31] Craig et al.[31] highlighted the importance of both childhood illness and lack of parental care in the development of unexplained symptoms. That lack of parental care should be a risk factor is unsurprising given its association with depression in later life. Using a population-based birth cohort study, Hotopf et al.[32] provided further evidence for the link between family ill health and unexplained abdominal pain in childhood. As well as being associated with unexplained physical symptoms in adulthood, persistent abdominal pain was a powerful predictor of adult psychiatric disorder. The developmental perspective has been reinforced by work focusing on the role of personality in somatisation. Many patients with chronic somatoform disorders also fulfil diagnostic criteria for personality disorders and this, in combination with the research on childhood antecedents, suggests that this method of communicating emotional distress may reflect an enduring personality trait.[33] Whether such traits influence the likelihood of acute somatised disorders becoming chronic has yet to be established. Alexithymia is a concept arising from psychodynamic theory that was introduced to describe an inability to resolve and express emotional conflict[34] with the consequent presentation of somatic symptoms. The majority of depressed patients presenting with somatic symptoms do, however, acknowledge psychological symptoms when questioned about them.[3,14] Indeed, there is a linear relationship between the number of physical symptoms and the number of psychological symptoms – the opposite of what would be expected under the alexithymia hypothesis. This suggests that somatisation does not reflect an inability to acknowledge psychological distress but that patients may feel this a more appropriate method of help-seeking.

Reinforcement and stigma

The stigmatisation of mental disorders, including depression, by both lay and medical populations is entrenched in Western culture and is a significant factor in the under-reporting of psychological problems.[35,36] Presenting with physical symptoms provides many advantages, which Goldberg and Bridges describe.[14] As well as affording a greater sense of legitimacy in adopting the sick role, we also have a system of sickness benefits and disability payments in which physical complaints are much more likely to be endorsed than psychological symptoms. The importance of stigma may also extend to a political level. Ware and Kleinman[37] described the escalation in the diagnosis of neurasthenia in Communist China. This occurred at a time when it was considered inappropriate to express oneself in terms of psychological distress as this was viewed as a moral or political statement. A diagnosis of neurasthenia (with its symptoms of fatigue, headaches and insomnia) in this context served as a form of protest about oppressive circumstances without risk of a political response.

Finally, the role of the doctor may also be a significant maintaining factor.[38] As a consequence of training that is essentially biological in orientation with an increasing emphasis on new technology, it is unsurprising that doctors will tend to focus on the identification and treatment of manifest organic disease, to the exclusion of psychosocial factors. Anxiety about missing a major physical illness (particularly in an environment of increasing litigation), and therapeutic impotence also contribute to reinforcing a narrow somatic model for symptoms.

Management of somatisation and depression

There are three steps that are essential for the effective management of somatic presentations of depression. Firstly, recognition of the presence of psychiatric disorder requires the taking of a full history that includes the patient's mental state and patients' own beliefs about their symptoms. The doctor also needs to be able to explore and respond to emotional cues which may indicate depression or anxiety. Secondly, central to management is the process of engaging the patient, making patients feel understood rather than rejected. This will involve broadening the agenda of the consultation and addressing psychosocial issues, as well as discussing the close relationship between physical and psychological symptoms. Whilst avoiding the erroneous implication that the reported symptoms are 'all in the mind', it is important to acknowledge the presence of emotional disorder and provide the patient with an explanation for their symptoms wherever possible. Basic examination and investigations are an essential part of management in primary care, but unless specifically indicated by signs of disease further investigations or secondary care referral should be avoided. Using investigations for reassurance may have a paradoxical effect, exacerbating anxiety about a 'missed' diagnosis. Finally, the discussion of specific treatments, antidepressants or brief psychological interventions, should reflect the explanation of the symptoms given to the patient.

Evidence for the benefit of treatments for somatisation in primary care is sparse, as intervention studies have taken place predominantly in specialist settings. However in a US primary care study,[39] Smith *et al.* demonstrated that this approach reduced health costs and improved physical function in patients with somatisation disorder. In the United Kingdom, Morriss *et al.* used a similar model in a training package for general practitioners that aimed to help somatising patients reattribute their symptoms to psychiatric disorder.[40] They found significant improvements in those patients who believed their symptoms were only partly physical in cause but not in those who believed their symptoms were entirely physical in nature. In an area that costs so much in terms of disability and healthcare resources, further studies are clearly necessary.

Conclusions

Somatisation is recognised as a common mechanism for expressing psychological distress and its universality is now well established. It is neither an abnormal or pathological means of presentation for healthcare and somatic symptoms appear to be as much a core component of depression as psychological symptoms. However, when depression manifests in this way, it is often neglected in the vain pursuit of a 'real' medical diagnosis, which may include inappropriate and potentially harmful investigations and treatments. Despite efforts to reduce the stigma associated with mental disorders, they remain tainted by a sense of moral failure. Depression is considered the result of a 'personality flaw' or a lack of 'willpower'. Unfortunately these misconceptions are reinforced by the narrow 'organic' focus of medical professionals and as a consequence we continue to fail many patients.

References

1. Kirmayer LJ, Young A. Culture and somatization: clinical, epidemiological, and ethnographic perspectives. *Psychosom Med* 1998;**60**:420–30.
2. Gureje O, Simon G, Üstün TB, Goldberg D. Somatization in cross-cultural perspective: a World Health Organization study in primary care. *Am J Psychiatry* 1997;**154**:989–95.
3. Simon GE, Von Korff M, Piccinelli M *et al.* An international study of the relation between somatic symptoms and depression. *N Engl J Med* 1999;**341**:1329–35.
4. Roberts BH, Norton NM. Prevalence of psychiatric illness in a medical outpatient clinic. *N Engl J Med* 1952;**245**:82.
5. Weich S, Lewis G, Donmall R, Mann A. Somatic presentation of psychiatric morbidity in general practice. *Br J Gen Practice* 1995;**45**:143–7.
6. Bridges KW, Goldberg DP. Somatic presentation of DSM-III psychiatric disorders in primary care. *J Psychosom Res* 1985;**29**:563–9.
7. Kirmayer LJ, Robbins JM, Dworkind M, Yaffe MJ. Somatization and the recognition of depression and anxiety in primary care. *Am J Psychiatry* 1993;**150**:734–41.
8. Escobar JI, Golding JM, Hough RL, *et al.* Somatisation in the community: relationship to disability and use of services. *Am J Public Health* 1987;**77**:837–40.
9. Smith GR. The course of somatization and its effects on utilization of health care resources. *Psychosomatics* 1994;**35**:263–67.
10. Fink P. The use of hospitalizations by persistent somatizing patients. *Psychol Med* 1992;**22**:173–80.
11. Paykel ES, Priest RG. Recognition and management of depression in general practice: consensus statement. *Br Med J* 1992;**305**:1198–202.
12. Katon W, Ries RK, Kleinman A. A prospective DSM-III study of 100 consecutive somatization patients. *Comprehen Psychiatry* 1984;**25**:305–14.
13. Murphy MR. Classification of the somatoform disorders. In: Bass C, ed. *Somatization: physical symptoms and psychological illness*. Oxford: Blackwell Scientific, 1990.
14. Goldberg DP, Bridges K. Somatic presentation of psychiatric illness in primary care setting. *J Psychosom Res* 1988;**32**:137–44.
15. Hickie I, Lloyd A, Wakefield D, Parker G. The psychiatric status of patients with the chronic fatigue syndrome. *Br J Psychiatry* 1990;**156**:534–40.
16. Drossman DA, McKee DC, Sandler RS *et al.* Psychosocial factors in the irritable bowel syndrome. *Gastroenterology* 1988;**95**:701–6.
17. Simon GE, Von Korff M. Somatization and psychiatric disorder in the NIMH Epidemiologic Catchment Area Study. *Am J Psychiatry* 1991;**148**:1494–500.
18. Katon W, Lin E, Von Korff M *et al.* Somatization: a spectrum of severity. *Am J Psychiatry* 1991;**148**:34–40.
19. Kroenke K, Price RK. Symptoms in the community: prevalence, classification, and psychiatric comorbidity. *Arch Intern Med.* 1993;**153**:2474–80.
20. Kirmayer LJ, Robbins JM. Three forms of somatization in primary care: prevalence, co-occurrence, and sociodemographic characteristics. *J Nervous Mental Dis* 1991;**179**:647–55.

21. Kroenke K, Spitzer RL, deGruy FV *et al*. Multisomatoform disorder. *Arch Gen Psychiatry* 1997;**54**:352–58.
22. Escobar JI. Overview of somatization: diagnosis, epidemiology, and management. *Psychopharmacol Bull* 1996;**32**:589–96.
23. Wool CA, Barsky AJ. Do women somatize more than men? Gender differences in somatization. *Psychosomatics* 1994;**35**:445–52.
24. Piccinelli M, Simon G. Gender and cross-cultural differences in somatic symptoms associated with emotional distress. An international study in primary care. *Psychol Med* 1997;**27**:433–44.
25. Cloninger CR, Sigvardsson S, Von Knorring AL, Bohman M. An adoption study of somatoform disorders. *Arch Gen Psychiatry* 1984;**41**:863–71.
26. Kendler KS, Walters EE, Truett KR *et al*. A twin-family study of self-report symptoms of panic-phobia and somatization. *Behavior Genetics* 1995;**25**:499–515.
27. Sharpe M, Bass C. Pathophysiological mechanisms in somatization. *Int Rev Psychiatry* 1992;**4**:81–97.
28. Drossman DA. Presidential address: 'Gastrointestinal illness and the biopsychosocial model.' *Psychosom Med*. 1998;**60**:258–67.
29. Mechanic D. The influence of mothers on their children's health attitudes and behavior. *Pediatrics* 1964;**33**:444–53.
30. Hartvig P, Sterner G. Childhood psychologic environmental exposure in women with diagnosed somatoform disorders. *Scand J Soc Med* 1985;**13**:153–57.
31. Craig TKJ, Boardman AP, Mills K *et al*. The South London somatisation study. I. Longitudinal course and the influence of early life experiences. *Br J Psychiatry* 1993;579–88.
32. Hotopf M, Carr S, Mayou R, Wadsworth MEJ, Wessely S. Why do children have chronic abdominal pain, and what happens to them when they grow up? *Br Med J* 1998;**316**:1196–200.
33. Bass C, Murphy M. Somatoform and personality disorders: syndromal comorbidity and overlapping developmental pathways. *J Psychosom Res* 1995;**39**:403–27.
34. Nemiah JC. A reconsideration of psychological specificity in psychosomatic disorders. *Psychother Psychosom* 1982;**38**:39–45.
35. Hudson JA. Mental illness made public: Ending the stigma? *Lancet* 1998;**352**:1060.
36. Porter R. Can the stigma of mental illness be changed? *Lancet* 1998;**352**:1049–50.
37. Ware N, Kleinman A. Culture and somatic experience – the social course of illness in neurasthenia and chronic fatigue syndrome. *Psychosom Med* 1992;**54**:546–60.
38. Kouyanou K, Pither CE, Rabe-Hesketh S, Wessely S. A comparative study of iatrogenesis, medication abuse, and psychiatric morbidity in chronic pain patients with and without medically unexplained symptoms. *Pain* 1998;**76**:417–26.
39. Smith GR Jr, Rost K, Kashner TM. A trial of the effect of a standardized psychiatric consultation on health outcomes and costs in somatizing patients. *Arch Gen Psychiatry* 1995;**52**:238–43.
40. Morriss RK, Gask L, Ronalds C *et al*. Clinical and patient satisfaction outcomes of a new treatment for somatized mental disorder taught to general practitioners. *Br J Gen Practice* 1999;**49**:263–67.

Male depression: stress and aggression as pathways to major depression

PER BECH

When Hamilton[1] made his first clinical validation study with his Hamilton Depression Rating Scale (HAM-D) the patients were all hospitalised for clinical depression and only males were included. In his next study[2] both males and females with clinical depression were included. He concluded: ... 'It is generally believed that women weep more readily than men, but there is little evidence that this is true in the case of depressive illness.' In his last study[3] he showed that the core symptoms of clinical depression are lowered mood, lack of interest and tiredness. According to the World Health Organization (WHO) classification system of mental disorders (ICD-10) it is a condition *sine qua non* for clinical (major) depression to have at least two of the three Hamilton symptoms.

Most epidemiological studies have shown that the ratio between females and males for clinical depression is 2:1, i.e. twice as many females as males. The only study in which this ratio of clinical depression is around 1 for females versus males is the Amish study on depression in which the percentage of males with major depression was 49%.[4] The subculture of the Amish people in Lancaster County, Pennsylvania, has the characteristic that males have grown up as if they were 'females', with a closer network than is found in other cultures and with no access to alcohol.

In his monograph on male depression, Real[5] has gathered evidence for the observation in the early stages that men tend to manifest depression differently to women. The pathway to the textbooks or ICD-10 symptoms seems to go via states of stress, aggression or alcohol abuse. This hypothesis has also been put forward by Rutz *et al.*[6]

In collaboration with the WHO Regional Office for Europe in

Copenhagen we have attempted to investigate the pathway to clinical depression when early symptoms of decreased positive wellbeing develop in life stress situations. Most health-related quality of life questionnaires have in common a general factor of positive psychological wellbeing.[7,8] From the Psychological General Well Being Scale (PGWB), the items in the WHO (five) Wellbeing Index, in correspondence to the 10 symptoms of depression (negative wellbeing), have been constructed and reduced from a 28-item version to 22 items,[9] 10 items[10] and finally to 5 items[11] (Table 2).

Table 2 Quality of life and depression: positive vs. negative wellbeing.

Positive wellbeing: PGWB items (WHO five)	Negative wellbeing: Major Depression Inventory (MDI)
• In good spirits	• Depressed mood
• Interested in things	• Lack of interests
• Active and vigorous	• Lack of energy
• Calm and relaxed	• Restless/subdued
• Fresh and rested	• Sleep disturbances
	• Decreased self-confidence
	• Guilt feelings
	• Life not worth living
	• Concentration difficulties
	• Appetite

In a Danish population study[12] including 1062 females and 1017 males, we found that 3.5% had a clinical (major) depression. When excluding this group with clinical depression we found that females scored significantly higher ($p \leq 0.05$) on the three core symptoms of depression while males scored higher on restlessness and suicidal ideas. However, in the sample of clinical (major) depression, no difference was seen in the symptoms.

In the Danish population study with the five items of positive wellbeing[13] we found no gender differences between males and females. The WHO (five) Wellbeing Index is transferred to a 0 to 100 scale in which 0 means the worst thinkable wellbeing and 100 means the best thinkable wellbeing. On this measure, the Danish normal population scored around 75 with no statistically significant difference between males and females or between younger and elderly people. Patients with major depression have a mean score of around 40 while patients seeking help for alcohol abuse have a score of around 55 with no difference between males and females.

In the study focusing on patients seeking help at the alcohol outpatient clinics in Copenhagen, the ratio between males and females was 2:1, i.e. twice as many males as females, or 387 versus 153.[14] Using the Symptom Checklist (SCL-90)[15] it was found that females scored significantly higher on items such as crying easily, headache, myalgia and people being unfriendly. Males score significantly higher on items such as aggression, never feeling close to another, and social anxiety.

Table 3 The Gotland Scale for Male Depression.

Depression factor	Distress factor
• Being burned out	• Being stressed
• Tiredness	• Aggressiveness
• Difficulty making decisions	• Restlessness
• Sleep problems	• Feeling of displeasure
• Hopelessness	• Overconsumption of alcohol
• Family history of depression or suicide	or related substances
	• Behaviour changes
	• Greater tendency to self-pitying

Table 3 shows the Gotland Scale for Male Depression, which has been developed by Rutz on the basis of his experiences gathered with his educational programme for family doctors on the island of Gotland, Sweden. Rutz demonstrated that the programme decreased the suicidal rate for females but not for males.[16]

The Gotland Scale for Male Depression was translated into Danish and analysed for internal validity concerning the two factors shown in Table 3. This validation study was carried out in the Alcohol Outpatient Clinic, Copenhagen ($n = 30$ males). The analysis of internal validity was performed with the Loevinger coefficient of homogeneity.[7,17] A coefficient of around 0.30 is estimated to be only doubtful while coefficients of around 0.40 are fully accepted when evaluating a scale for homogeneity and unidimensionality. The results showed that the depression factor had a Loevinger coefficient of 0.32 while the distress factor was 0.39, indicating that the total score of the distress factor is a sufficient statistic.

The main argument for using traditional depression instruments to show that twice as many females compared to males are suffering from depression is postnatal depression. This condition has its onset weeks after childbirth. Immediately after the delivery the depressive reaction often is referred to as 'baby blues', which is seen in 50% of the mothers while postnatal depression is seen in 10%. However, 'baby blues' as seen in the father is now under examination, using the Gotland Male Depression Scale as well as the WHO (five) Wellbeing Index as measures.

The most famous example of male depression is probably the case of Ernest Hemingway. His special gift was his attempt to give his readers insight into an uncompromisingly male psyche. However, his own periods of depression were masked by alcohol abuse, restlessness and aggression. He committed suicide in 1961, just before antidepressants became available.[18]

Acknowledgement

I would like to acknowledge the help of those colleagues with whom I collaborated.

References

1. Hamilton M. A rating scale for depression. *J Neurol Neurosurg Psychiatry* 1960;**23**:56–62.
2. Hamilton M. Development of a rating scale for primary depressive illness. *Br J Soc Clin Psychol* 1967;**6**:278–96.
3. Hamilton M. Frequency of symptoms in melancholia (depressive illness). *Br J Psychiatry* 1989;**154**:201–6.
4. Egeland JA, Hostetter AM, Eshleman SK. Amish Study. III: The impact of cultural factors on diagnosis of bipolar illness. *Am J Psychiatry* 1983;**140**:67–71.
5. Real T. *I Don't Want to Talk About It: overcoming the secret legacy of male depression.* New York: Fireside Books, 1998.
6. Rutz W, von Knorring L, Pihlgren H *et al.* Prevention of male suicides: lessons from Gotland study. *Lancet* 1995;**345**:524.
7. Bech P. *Rating Scales for Psychopathology, Health Status and Quality of Life: a compendium on documentation in accordance with the DSM-III-R and WHO systems.* New York: Springer-Verlag, 1993.
8. Pukrop R, Steinmeyer EM. Item analysis of quality of life instruments in depression and schizophrenia. *Pharmacopsychiatry* 1997;**30**:208–9.
9. Bradley C, ed. *Handbook of Psychology and Diabetes: a guide to psychological measurement in diabetes research and practice.* London: Harwood, 1994.
10. Bech P, Gudex C, Johansen KS. The WHO (ten) Wellbeing Index: validation in diabetes. *Psychother Psychom* 1996;**65**:183–90.
11. Heun R, Burkart M, Maier W, Bech P. Internal and external validity of the WHO Well-Being Scale in the elderly general population. *Acta Psychiatr Scand* 1999;**99**:171–8.
12. Olsen LR, Noerholm V, Bech P. Major Depression Inventory: a Danish normal population study (in preparation, 1999).
13. Rasmussen NA, Noerholm V, Bech P *et al.* Psychological General Wellbeing Schedule: a Danish normal population study (in preparation, 1999).
14. Zierau F, Olsen LR, Bech P. The Hopkins Symptom Checklist (SCL-90) in alcohol abuse disorders (in preparation, 1999).
15. Bech P, Allerup P, Maier W *et al.* The Hamilton scales and the Hopkins Symptom Checklist (SCL-90): a cross-national validity study in patients with panic disorders. *Br J Psychiatry* 1992;**160**:206–11.
16. Rutz W. Improvement of care for people suffering from depression: the need for comprehensive education. *Int Clin Psychopharmacol* 1999;**14**(Suppl 3): S27–33.
17. Mokken RJ. *A Theory and Procedure of Scale Analysis, with Applications in Political Research.* Paris: Mouton, 1971.
18. Reynolds MS. *Hemingway: the final years.* New York: Norton, 1999.

Improving the recognition and monitoring of depressive conditions: implications for suicide prevention

WOLFGANG RUTZ

Introduction

The situation regarding research on suicide prevention and, consequent to that, the development of suicide prevention strategies, appears today somewhat confusing. Different risk variables for suicides have been found: sociological factors such as unemployment, biological factors such as heredity for depression, psychological factors such as loss of identity and helplessness as well as existential factors regarding anomie and existential emptiness.

However, none of these findings is consistent. From country to country different factors appear to have a different impact, in different societies or regarding different groups with suicidal behaviour. Single suicidal attempters, or multiple suicidal attempters, are differing suicidal populations at risk, as well as groups with different risk-taking lifestyles all at different ages. Cultural factors may also play a role concerning the impact of societal change as well as the phenomenology of psychopathological dysfunction. Depressive suicide causing ideation may be as bad a sin in some societies (for example, in ex-pietistic Swedish regions) as the fear of genital retraction into the body may be in other cultures, (for example, in India). Morbidity as depression, anxiety states or personality disorders, as well as different types of risk-taking, life-shortening, aggressive suicidal behaviour have to be taken into account – and they present uniquely in different societies. As in one country unemployment may mainly cause helplessness, depression and suicide, so in another society it can be stress due to work overload having these same effects.

67

One of the most consistent findings, however, is that suicide is committed in a psychopathological condition or in the course of a psychiatric disorder. Even these psychopathological conditions, however, have to be seen as a result of a multifactorial process where biological, sociological, psychological and existential factors in interaction, and mutual reinforcement lead to disorder and dysfunction. As an example, we can find depression to be one of the common final pathways and a condition *sine qua non* in the majority of all suicides. This has to be seen as a process from a more generic and complex aetiological background to a quite specific suicide-provoking condition. The longer the process lasts, the more specific the suicide preventive or curative intervention has to be. In the last phase, for example, a specific antidepressive treatment may be needed. In addition to what has been said, it has to be seen that abusive and risk-taking behaviour, such as drug abuse in women, or 'psychopathic' aggressive and/or suicidal acting-out or alcoholism in males and adolescents, in many cases is related to or covering helplessness, related depression and anxiety.

To detect and treat depressive conditions as the main common final pathway in the process of suicide was the aim of the Gotland Study. The study was implemented as an educational programme during the beginning of the 1980s, evaluated until the beginning of the 1990s and followed up with maintenance education until 1998. The study, its successes and shortcomings, illustrates the possibilities, as well as the limitations, that the medical psychiatric systems have to face when taking their obligatory responsibility for the improvement of treatment and monitoring of psychiatric morbidity, which, in the vast majority of completed suicides, can be found as the direct causative factor to the suicidal act. Few suicides are committed in a 'philosophical' way, where realistic and cognitively non-disturbed judgements could be made by the suicidal person. Most suicides are consistently committed during a state of psychopathological condition with subsequent depressive distortion, dysfunctional perception and loss of reality.

The Gotland Study

In spite of its apparent life quality and beauty, the Swedish island of Gotland, with 60 000 inhabitants, being a psychiatric sector and an epidemiologically 'transparent' laboratory, with a society in dramatic social transition, was during the 1970s one of the 'black areas' with respect to Sweden. The suicide rate on the island was amongst the highest in Sweden, well above urban figures, characterised by a high rate of often violent suicide also in females. One of the lowest prescription levels of specific antidepressants in Sweden existed on the island but was 'compensated' for by a high overprescription of sedative, anxiolytic and hypnotic drugs.

In this alarming situation, initiatives for an educational activity came from the general practitioners eager to assist their helpless patients. To assist the general practitioners and to counter the island's problems regarding depression and suicide, the local psychiatric department, together with the Swedish Committee for Prevention and Treatment of Depressions (PTD Committee), began an educational programme on depression in primary health care. This comprehensive and structured programme, given twice over two days, was offered during a two-year period to all general practitioners on Gotland. It covered most aspects of the detection and monitoring of depressive disorders and all but one general practitioner participated. The programme was carried out in a somewhat luxurious hotel environment and boarding-house situation over a two-day period. The one night in between gave opportunity for interaction, discussion and the sharing of personal clinical and private experiences, lectures as well as video presentations, and case discussions. Participants had the possibility to influence the programme, highlighting omissions, and were given the educational material in written form, in order to teach their own teams. The problem of depression, its detection and monitoring, was addressed in an integrative and synoptic way. The process of becoming depressed and consequently suicidal – and recovering from it – presented opportunity for a demanding multidisciplinary and multimodal intervention. The sometimes crucial and inevitable need for psychopharmacological treatment was presented as well as the need for psychotherapeutic follow up and support in a process-related way. Psychotherapy and pharmacological therapy were presented as complementary approaches rather than as alternative strategies. Consequently a split between 'endogenicity' and 'exogenicity' was avoided as well as the dichotomy between psychodynamic-psychosocial considerations and biological views, using a stress-vulnerability model. The need for process and integrative thinking was underlined regarding the importance of taking into consideration multifactorial causalities and the need to act in a process related manner. This 'holistic' approach was reflected in our attempts not to present depression as a distinctly definable limited nosological entity attached with different co-morbidities, but including also anxiety, drug abuse, alcoholism, temporary depressive personality changes and different types of destructive behaviour as symptoms often related to and caused by depression.

Presented in this structured and holistic way, the educational programme was highly appreciated and led to a significant improvement of the general practitioners' capacity to diagnose, to treat and to monitor depressive conditions. During the three years following the programme, which was the time of the maximum effects, a cascade of different results related to the education and interrelated to each other could be noted. Referrals for depression to the local psychiatric institution, as well as the amount of sick leave for depressive and apathetic conditions on Gotland, dropped by more than 50%. The amount of inpatient care for depressive conditions at the local psychiatric clinic dropped by 30%, and suicides decreased by about two-thirds. The prescribing of antidepressants increased from less then 50% of the Swedish average to above 80%. However, sedative, anxiolytic and hypnotic prescriptions decreased by 30% compared to Sweden, thus normalising the earlier overprescribing. Three years after the programme, as a consequence of the diagnosis of recurrent depressive conditions, the prescribing of lithium increased also by 30%. However, these changes were strictly time related since, after a decade, the changes returned to about baseline values and the need for maintained and repeated education became apparent. Re-education started in the beginning of the 1990s and updating follow-up education programmes were given until 1998 at about two-yearly intervals.

A special cost-benefit calculation showed that the costs of the educational programme were about SKr 400 000, resulting in savings for society of up to SKr 150 000 000 during the three-year period of maximum effect, due to reduced morbidity, reduced suicide mortality, reduced inpatient care and reduced drug expenses.

On scrutinising the suicide-preventive effect of this education programme, additional results were found. The decrease in suicide following the programme was significant and led, during some of the follow-up years, to the lowest rate of suicide found in Gotland and in Sweden. This was expected due to the fact that the programme had aimed to improve the capacity of general practitioners to recognise depression and it was already known that the most decisive suicides are often those caused by depression. What was not expected, however, was that these positive changes were only found in the group of female suicides and that male suicide rates continued almost unchanged. Apparently the programme, directed to general practitioners and focused on improving quality of recognition and monitoring of depression, had not improved male suicide rates in Gotland. Most male suicides were committed without any contact with the medical system. In the few cases where such contact with psychiatry did exist and/or primary healthcare took place, the future suicide subjects were classified as personality disturbed, sociopathic behaving, abusers and often considered impossible to treat due to improper behaviour, 'psychopatic' acting-out, aggressiveness and/or lack of compliance and motivation. In contrast to the few female suicides in Gotland during the 1990s (who, in the majority, were known to the medical system), the majority of the many male suicides were known to police, to tax authorities or social authorities responsible for alcoholics, if indeed they were in contact with society at all.

In the mid-1990s there were hardly any female suicides in Gotland. Facing the still high male suicide rate, however, the follow-up educational programmes were given an increased focus on male depression and suicidal behaviour, describing male acting-out, destructive risk-taking, abuse and non-compliance. After this, for the first time, even male suicides appeared to decrease.

Another recent find showed that the seasonality in patterns of suicides in Gotland, which was quite noticeable during the 1980s, had significantly decreased during the 1990s. This may be due to the fact that depressions are seasonal and that the situation in Gotland before the educational project was one of underdiagnosis and undertreatment of depression.

Conclusions

Education aimed at the better recognition and monitoring of depression-related conditions in primary care seems to prevent suicide. The data show the importance of general practitioners as the first line in the diagnosis and treatment of depression. However, there still exists in many parts of Europe an incapacity of primary care to take this responsibility. Experiences with educational programmes from the United Kingdom, Hungary, the Baltic states, the United States and Canada, underline that education presented in a way similar to the Gotland model may increase the specificity of pharmacological treatment of depression, by increased prescribing of antidepressives as well as lithium, and decreases the prescribing of unspecific sedatives, hypnotics and anxiolytics. These findings are supported by increasing experiences regarding the probable suicide-preventive effect of antidepressive medication.

However, the mere improvement in pharmacological treatment of depression might not be enough. Certainly, in many European countries, the improved detection and treatment of depression have led to a more adequate pharmacological supply of antidepressants in the population, probably decreasing suicidality. In Sweden, for example, the increase in antidepressive prescriptions by 200% during the 1990s was accompanied by a decrease in suicidality by 25%. However, in Gotland, where the increase of antidepressive prescriptions by 300% during the 1990s was complemented by educational follow-up programmes on depression and suicide to general practitioners every second year, the concomitant decrease in suicides was 50%. Thus, educational programmes, focusing both on the need for diagnosis and medication, indicate such programmes need to be integrated in a holistic context of sociopsychological support and existential reflection, as has been done in Gotland, in order to have the optimum effect.

Depressive and suicidal males behave typically in a manner different from females, most often showing 'atypical' depressive symptomatology. They are seldom in contact with the medical system and – if they casually request help – are often not recognised, refused or not treated effectively. In Gotland, a scale focusing on the typical 'atypical' male depressive symptoms has been developed, presenting the male depressive picture of lowered stress

71

tolerance, acting-out, aggressiveness, low impulse control, irritability, indecisiveness, abuse tendencies, temporary 'antisocial' behaviour with male heredity for suicide, depression and abuse as typical features. This scale is based on scientific and clinical experience and has for some years been tested successfully as a screening instrument to find depression in males amongst those who are not complaining about or showing typical depressive symptoms, but who are in contact with primary care, other medical care, in the work places or other social settings. At this time, this scale is undergoing scientific evaluation and validation. Since this Gotland Scale for Male Depression' has been taught as a screening instrument to the Gotlandian primary healthcare system and presented in the Gotlandian mass media, a decrease in male suicides in Gotland has been found.

The concept of male depression and suicide is gaining scientific interest in increasing contexts. However, due to the fact that most male depressive suicidal subjects are not in contact with any medical system, approaches have to be developed to reach them through different sectors of society, the workplace, trade unions, social networks, families and friends, as well as the mass media.

Summing up, the indications for regional underdiagnosis of depression and consequently for the expected efficiency of educational interventions as described in relation to the Gotland model, are as follow:

- underprescription of specific antidepressive medication;
- overprescription of unspecific sedative, anxiolytic and hypnotic medications;
- high frequency of sick leave for depressive and depression-related conditions;
- a high rate of especially intentional, drastic suicides;
- populations with the most vulnerable risk groups exposed to changes, including elderly, rural populations and adolescents non-related males;
- populations where societal changes seem to be specifically pathogenic and suicidogenic with regard to sociological and cultural patterns of the society;
- unemployment, which, might have a different on impact depression in the Protestant societies of western Europe compared to some of the African cultures;
- social exclusion, which may have a greater impact on depression and suicide in some African countries than in western Europe;
- the existence of clear seasonal patterns in the suicide rate in a region, which might be proof of depression-related, undetected, untreated but preventable suicidality.

Present challenges and future perspectives

In HEALTH21, Health For All in the 21st Century, WHO has identified health as a basic human right, demanding participation and accountability by all sectors of society from governmental to local level, in approaches oriented to the family, community and primary healthcare and involving different partners and settings in society. With regard to dramatically decreasing life expectancy, especially in the Eastern European countries in transition, and especially in rural areas and mostly in males, we are facing one of the greatest challenges for public health concerns in Europe today.

Those societies at special risk are in need of concerted help, including scientific and evidence-based support, given in a comprehensive way, integrating psychological, sociological, existential and biological methods of suicide prevention as described in this article. Looking at the Europe of today, some countries can be found where suicide rate is decreasing, with a decrease also in the prevalence of depression and depression-related conditions. However, other countries can be found with an increased prevalence of depression but which, in spite of this, show a decreasing or stable rate of suicide. In Eastern Europe, especially, we find today a situation of a dramatically increasing rate of suicide and depression in need of urgent, acute and rapid intervention. Probably one of the specific factors differentiating these countries from each other is the easy and ready access to detection, treatment and monitoring of depression and anxiety – not only in their typical forms, but also for depressive people with self-medicating abuse, depressive risk-taking behaviour, and suicidal or self-destructive acting-out lifestyles and habits.

The dramatic increase in suicide in Eastern Europe is declared to be one of the main calls for action facilitated by WHO. It has to be seen in the context of a parallel increase of other helplessness and depression-related morbidity and mortality in those countries in which there is an increase in deaths due to risk-taking behaviour, death by external causes through violence and accidents, mortality due to abusive destructive behaviour and mortality due to cardiovascular diseases. Depression-related suicidality and other stress-related morbidity and consequent mortality in general are a main cause of the decreasing life expectancy in Eastern Europe and have to be tackled together as a cluster of conditions in their help-and hopelessness-related context. Besides strategies for decreasing stress, increasing social coherence and stress-coping ability in a society, sociological interventions directed at employment, social identity and dignity are in demand – as well as measures to decrease access to alcohol and access to known methods of suicide. However, those strategies are often hard to realise. In this situation at least the improvement of access to proper detection and monitoring of depressive conditions and depression related suicide based on sound scientific and empirical evidence seems to be realistic and feasible.

Thus, one of the challenges today – being both possible and also the responsibility of the medical system – is to improve the detection and treatment of depression as a psychiatric disorder leading most frequently to fatal suicidal consequences. To achieve this, education on depression and suicide is needed for general practitioners and also for other professionals belonging to primary healthcare teams. This education should be continuous, obligatory, and presented in a motivating and learning-facilitating way.

Undetected male depression and suicide and their underdiagnosis and undertreatment might be the explanation for the paradox that females twice as often as males are diagnosed as depressive, but males for some reason are committing suicide two to five times more often than females. To reach those males is especially demanding. We know that it is the male population that is most vulnerable to societal change and transition, reacting with increased mortality due to stress-related and helplessness-related conditions including suicide, as described above. To diagnose the breakdown of stress-coping ability that we call depression, and that might appear differently in males and females, we need new and specific diagnostic instruments to find these males, in order to offer them a proper therapeutic approach with which they are able to cope and that in turn treats them.

A still greater challenge is to focus on another paradox in public health today, namely that males show a morbidity that is much lower than that in females, but their mortality is so much higher and their life expectancy so much shorter than in the female population. This, in spite of the absence of registered and known disease. Strategies needed here involve not only the development of programmes enabling stress coping and stress-management capacities, but also the need to develop cognitive strategies and therapeutic modules to teach male populations at risk to show the strength to show weakness and helplessness in time, in order to get help and treatment before it is too late. To integrate this into comprehensive educational programmes, according to the Gotland programme, could be one of the future models to achieve further impact with this approach.

Depression and General Practice

Overview

This section deals with various aspects of primary care management of depression. Up to 30% of primary care attendees suffer from depression. For various reasons diagnosis is not always straightforward, often because the patient may not present with classical symptoms. For instance, it has been estimated that in 25% of cases of back pain, the underlying cause is depression. Once diagnosed, depression brings special burdens to the general practitioner, not least because of problems with the patient's drug management such as ineffective or inappropriate treatment or defaulting on treatment; problems that conspire to make the patient a regular attendee at the surgery.

In recent years, emphasis has been placed on team working and ensuring that each team member is adequately trained for the task. In this respect PriMHE, a UK national association specialising in primary care mental health education, is playing a pivotal role in the United Kingdom. In the United States Kaiser Permanente has developed a primary care evidence-based managed package of care for people with depression that involves the use of algorithms. It is also based on case identification and the notion that 'you cannot improve unless you manage' and 'you can't manage unless you measure', which is predicated on having information systems that allow us to do that.

Depression causes special suffering as it affects, centrally and directly, the whole quality of the patient's life. A glimpse of what it is like to be a sufferer and the effects it has on all the family, especially when more than one member of that family is affected, is reported here.

National Service Framework for Mental Health

In early October 1999 an important European Conference on Mental Health and Social Inclusion was held in Finland. It was attended by the ministers of health from all over Europe as well as the Director-General of WHO Dr Gro Harlem Brundtland. The aim of the meeting was to raise the profile of mental health in Europe making it a key objective for governments, national organisations and local agencies. In keeping with Target 6 of the WHO health for all policy, each participating country was encouraged to make mental health a priority issue. At the meeting the English Minister of Health stated that her country had already risen to that challenge and had developed a National Service Framework, which focused on the mental health needs of adults in the working-age bracket, and set standards that will be used to:

- drive up the quality of local mental health services;
- reduce wide variations;
- and measure performance.

A brief summary of the National Service Framework, produced by PriMHE, and based on the Department of Health's original document, is reproduced here with their kind permission.

Depression and general practice

SIR DENIS PEREIRA GRAY

Depression is a condition of great general interest. It is common, it is serious, and few other conditions so affect the quality of life.

> Of all 'the common ills that flesh is heir to', depression causes special suffering as it affects, centrally and directly, the whole quality of patients' lives. Of all the diseases to miss, this is the one that touches the general practitioner's professional ethos the most because, of all doctors, generalists relate to the whole person and not just to the sum of the patient's component parts.[1]

It is particularly rewarding professionally.

Kipling's six headings provide a framework: 'what, where, when and how, and why and who.'

What?

Depression is relatively simple to describe in clinical terms, but complex to measure scientifically. It is a lowering of mood beyond the range of ups and downs encountered in normal life and sustained over time and to such a degree that the person's quality of life is significantly impaired.

Defining it scientifically is more difficult and has led to international agreement that it is present only when certain symptoms are present in agreed combinations, for example the International Classification of Disease, ICD-10,[2] or the American equivalent DSM.[3] Such agreements have been fundamental to carrying out meaningful comparisons and have formed the basis of research on all the treatments. They are much less useful in clinical practice and especially in primary care.

Diagnosis by questionnaire is routine in research: it is less easy and appropriate in clinical care. How often does one see a psychiatrist's report that gives a Beck, a Hospital Anxiety and Depression Scale (HADS) or Hamilton, score? In practice, in both primary and secondary care, depression is a clinical diagnosis. There is no blood test or investigation that helps. How common it is depends on the questionnaire used, and instruments like the HADS rate most British populations as having about 5-7.5% with major depression, and up to three times this with less severe forms of depression.

In research studies, general practitioners diagnose depression much less often[4]. This is a cause of great discussion in both academic general practice and psychiatry. Clearly there is a skills deficit of some magnitude.

Equally, the research method rested on the analysis of single consultations and general practice depends on a series of contacts. Secondly, outcomes from general practice care tend to be better than expected[5] as general practitioner reassurance, support or 'enablement'[6] are undervalued in the research literature.[7]

Where?

Not only is depression very common, which in itself makes it logical to manage in primary care, but the symptoms with which it is associated are very common too. Fatigue, for example, is extremely common as a presenting symptom. But fatigue can also be associated with anaemia, the presentation of diabetes, or malignant disease and, once in a general practitioner's professional lifetime, it may be the presentation of Addison's disease. The fascination of being a clinical generalist is that one has to handle all these possibilities all at the same time.

Thus it is possible and desirable for psychiatrists to lay down protocols for the investigation of depression in psychiatric practice, but it is not possible for them to do so in general practice. The probabilities are different: so the investigations need to be different too. Thus arranging a blood count and testing for diabetes may be entirely appropriate at the same consultation when a generalist is first examining the mental state.

Personal significance

A further fascinating dimension is the patient's point of view. In no other branch of medicine is the perception of the patient of greater importance than in general practice. First, the very nature of primary care, i.e. offering an open access service off the street, makes primary physicians the world over interested in and sensitive to the many cultural features of society. What may signify health in one culture may signify disease in another. The understanding as to why the patient has consulted at all, and why now, are core features of the generalist's consultation that may be of very little interest to a specialist. Patients also have hopes and fears that they bring to the consultation.

Generalists have to identify these and work with them. If a patient has a fixed idea about the nature of his or her problem and how it should be treated, whether or not the general practitioner agrees, this has to be taken into account. Generalists are thus concerned with what they call 'personal significance'[8]. This is a clinical amalgam of concepts like health beliefs, culture, class, creed, symptom attribution[9] as well as an understanding of family dynamics. Many consultations in primary care arise because members of the patient's family have concerns.[10]

Where depression is diagnosed and treated is clear. Watts and Watts[11] in their book *Psychiatry in General Practice* in 1952, reported that 18% of consultations in general practice were for conditions diagnosed as essentially emotional. Shepherd *et al.* years later confirmed this.[12]

It is clear that the mass of patients suffering from depression present in general practice. Over 90% of depressives are treated solely in general practice and fewer than 10% are referred to any specialised service. As Shepherd[12] wrote, the task is not how to fit the family doctor into the mental health services, but how to fit the mental health services into family medicine. This is quite reasonable as long as the primary care clinicians are highly skilled generalists and can translate physical complaints and social problems into psychological terms when necessary. As another internationally renowned psychiatrist, Sir Denis Hill,[13] in 1969 wrote: 'The family doctor's task is a difficult one and family doctors need to become the most comprehensively educated doctors.' Alas, even in 1999, the period of training for most generalists in their own discipline remains as little as 12 months.

Another advantage of managing depression in general practice is the chronicity of the condition. Lloyd *et al.*[14] showed the long-term outcome. 'Once depressed always depressed' is an overstatement, but it is best to regard depression as often a chronic condition.

One interesting and important issue is the presentation by patients of what they believe are physical symptoms, when in the doctor's mind the origin is psychological. This so-called 'somatisation' is a considerable intellectual challenge and also is emotionally demanding. Many such patients are hard to convince and the medical generalist always has to consider whether or not there could be a physical cause. The key issue is cancer, which can have a variety of presentations especially in its earlier phases. Somatising patients who are depressed, frequently, not just fear, but firmly believe they have got cancer.

The generalist thus has to work in at least two dimensions simultaneously: i.e. physical and psychological medicine. Blood tests may have to be done to exclude what the patient fears, whilst the therapeutic relationship is built up to provide care for the underlying depression.

General practice is centrally important in the detection and treatment of depression (Box 2).

Box 2   General practice in the detection and treatment of depression.

- General practice is the most logical place to diagnose depression.
- Patients do not go to the doctor with diseases, but with symptoms.[15] Only a generalist can optimally sort out what is physical, what is psychological, and what is social.[16] Furthermore, as these are not discrete categories, then the key is really assessing how much the physical dimension is involved, how much the psychological dimension, and how much the social when all three are factors – and all at once.
- The generalist is more likely to be briefed about the relevant factors that alter the probability of a diagnosis of depression. For example, a family history of depression is more likely to be known by a general practitioner than by a specialised service. Indeed, the general practitioner may often have known and treated the family member concerned.
- A previous history of depression is critical and having the long-term medical record greatly improves diagnosis, especially since recent research has established that depression is so often a chronic disease.[14]
- Psychiatric care is still stigmatised. General practice offers a non-stigmatising, easily accessible source of care to the whole population.

Why?

There are two main reasons why people become depressed: genetic and environmental factors. Both are of special importance to family doctors.

- Familial reasons
  Depression runs in families, a fact that is soon very obvious to family doctors. It is probable that a gene for depression will be identified in the next few years.
- Environmental reasons
  Secondly, depression is associated with altered relationships. General practitioners are especially interested in relationships and have on average the longest doctor-patient relationships of any kind of doctor. Twenty-five year doctor-patient relationships are not uncommon in general practice. Relationship analysis and understanding is necessary in caring for people suffering from depression.

When?

Depression is well known to be more likely to occur in certain situations, all of which are commonly seen in general practice and some of which are exclusively managed in general practice. These so-called special forms of depression are better regarded as special situations in which depression is particularly common.

- Postviral infection
- Premenstrual
- Postnatal
- Post-bereavement
- Seasonal affective disorder (SAD)
- Loss of an existing or expected relationship
- Having a handicapped child or an unfulfilling marriage.

Two points stand out: first the obvious physical form of some of these triggers, e.g. viral infections and the hormonal influences of childbirth and menstruation. Secondly, that any significant loss of relationship can act as a trigger.

How?

Depression can be treated in several different ways. The two keys are talking and drugs. Most British patients have a preference for talking as treatment and fear drugs as many believe they are addictive.[17]

In United Kingdom general practice the mainstays of treatment are: reassurance, support and antidepressant medication. The first is little understood, but important. Many depressed patients fear that they are going to go mad, and confident, sensitive, supportive reassurance can go a long way in fostering recovery (as well as compliance). Specific talking therapies such as cognitive behavioural therapy have been shown to be effective, as has interpersonal psychotherapy. They are not easily available in the United Kingdom National Health Service (NHS).

The proportion of patients with mental health problems treated in primary care is about 90%, mainly depression, anxiety states and drug addiction. This means that general practice is the main form of mental health service in the NHS. Re-categorisation is needed to make this clearer as some official documents use the term 'mental health services' as synonymous with the specialised mental health services.

In the past, tricyclic antidepressants were the mainstay for drug therapy, but more and more general practitioners are now using selective serotonin-reuptake inhibitors (SSRIs) (Ferguson, Medical Director, PPA, personal communication, 1999). This is because they are easier to use, have fewer side effects and allow patients to drive. They also protect general practitioners against accusations that they are using inadequate doses.

One difficulty that arises is the choice of dose. Here there is a tension between two disciplines: general practice and psychiatry. For example, most academic research psychiatrists write about the importance of using the doses that performed best in randomised controlled trials. This is reasonable and is the normal approach in medicine. However, depression is a disease that arouses strong feelings amongst patients, many of whom do not want to take drugs at all and, if they do, they want the lowest possible dose. General practitioners tend to use lower doses and rely on reaching agreement with the patient as to what is the best dose for each individual person. A second argument is that the right dose is enough, i.e. what is needed to get each individual patient better. Psychiatrists tend to favour the group approach, the general practitioners the individual approach.

Psychiatrists have the weight of the volume of published studies on their side; on the other hand, general practitioners performed well in one of the few prospective randomised controlled trials comparing psychiatrists with their favoured doses against routine general practitioner care.[5] No benefit in outcome was found from specialist care. Thus 'routine general practitioner care' is more valuable than has been thought[7] and may be effective as it includes considerable reassurance and support, sensible practical advice, a usually familiar face (the personal doctor) and a shoulder to cry on. Howie et al. called the success factor of routine general practitioner care 'enablement.'[6] Patients are more satisfied with general practice than with either hospital inpatients or outpatients.[18]

Issues for the future

It is probable that depression is getting commoner. One difficulty in interpretation is that of improved diagnostic methods and greater awareness, for example through the 'Defeat Depression' campaign of the Royal Colleges of Psychiatrists and General Practitioners. Nevertheless, the current consensus is that the incidence and prevalence are both rising. In particular, there is evidence that younger generations are suffering from depression proportionally more than older generations. It is not yet known why this should be, but WHO has already stated that it foresees depression becoming one of the main health problems in the world in the short-term future.

Some of the features of modern developed societies may be contributing to the increase, such as the lessening of sustained relationships (especially at home and at work), greater pace of change and better dissemination of information. The last may seem surprising, but informed patients are increasingly worried patients. Paternalism is now outmoded, but it is sometimes forgotten that its purpose was to shield patients from unpleasant information. Passing on more and more information, especially about risks and complications, is leading to much better informed and more autonomous patients, but also more and more people burdened with new and unwelcome knowledge. We are entering an Age of Anxiety.

Conclusion

Depression is one of the most important diseases of our time. It is common and getting commoner. It is serious in that it severely affects the quality of life and it is associated with a worrying number of deaths from suicide. It is especially important in general practice, where over 90% of patients are diagnosed and treated. Depression is most efficiently managed in primary care as both the familial features and the environmental features associated with its cause are best known and assessed there.

Depression is usually treatable. Although up to a third of patients may not respond to standard antidepressant drugs in conventional doses, a change of medication may work and other treatments are available.

Box 3 The keys to improving care in general practice in the future

- Longer training for clinical generalists. Twelve months in the specialty of general practice is simply not enough.
- Steps need to be taken to allow generalists to lengthen their consultations. Even though the NHS general practitioner has on average 'Forty-seven minutes a year for the patient',[19] this is still not enough.
- The greater adoption of the personal list system of practice organisation has been shown to increase continuity of care[20] and also satisfaction by patients.[21]

The prescribing of antidepressants in general practice in the NHS reveals dramatic increases. This confirms that general practice is increasingly responding to need.

References

1. Pereira Gray DJ. Depression in general practice. In: *RCGP Members' Reference Book 1992.* pp.205–11. London: Sterling Publications, 1992.
2. World Health Organization. *The ICD-10 Classification of Mental and Behavioural Disorders: clinical descriptions and diagnostic guidelines.* Geneva: World Health Organization, 1992.
3. American Psychiatric Association. *Diagnostic and Statistical Manual of Mental Disorders.* DSM-III-R. Washington, DC: American Psychiatric Association, 1987.
4. Freeling P, Rao BM, Paykel ES *et al.* Unrecognised depression in general practice. *BMJ* 1985;**290**:1880–3.
5. Scott AI, Freeman CP. Edinburgh Primary Care Depression Study: treatment outcomes, patient satisfaction and cost after 16 weeks. *BMJ* 1992;**304**:883–87.

6. Howie JGR, Heaney DJ, Maxwell M. *Measuring Quality in General Practice. Occasional Paper 75*. London: Royal College of General Practitioners.
7. Friedli K, King MB, Lloyd M, Horder J. Randomised controlled assessment of non-directive psychotherapy versus routine general-practitioner care. *Lancet* 1997;**350**:1662–65.
8. Sweeney KG, MacAuley D, Pereira Gray DJ. Personal significance: the third dimension. *Lancet* 1998;**351**:134–36.
9. Kessler D, Lloyd K, Lewis G, Pereira Gray D. Cross sectional study of symptom attribution and recognition of depression and anxiety in primary care. *BMJ* 1999;**318**:436–40.
10. Bailey AJM. Home visiting: the part played by the 'intermediary'. *J Royal Coll Gen Practit* 1979;**29**:137–42.
11. Watts CAH and Watts BM. *Psychiatry in General Practice*. London: J&A Churchill, 1952.
12. Shepherd M, Cooper M, Brown AC, Kalton G. *Psychiatric Illness in General Practice*. London: Oxford University Press, 1966.
13. Hill D. *Psychiatry in Medicine. Retrospect and prospect*. London: Nuffield Provincial Hospitals Trust, 1969.
14. Lloyd KR, Jenkins R, Mann A. Long-term outcome of patients with neurotic illness in general practice. *BMJ* 1996;**313**:26–8.
15. Helman CG. Disease versus illness in general practice. *J Royal Coll Gen Practit* 1981;**31**:548–52.
16. Pereira Gray DJ. The care of the handicapped child in general practice. Gold Medal Essay 1969. *Trans Hunterian Soc* 1971;**28**,121–75.
17. Paykel ES, Hart D, Priest RG. Changes in public attitudes to depression during the 'Defeat Depression' campaign. *Br J Psychiatry* 1998;**173**:519–22.
18. Jowell R, Witherspoon S, Brook L. *British Social Attitudes*, p.17. Aldershot: Gower, 1990.
19. Pereira Gray DJ. Forty-seven minutes a year for the patient. [Editorial.] *Br J Gen Pract* 1998;**48**:1816–7.
20. Roland M, Mayor V, Morris R. Factors associated with achieving continuity of care in general practice. *J Royal Coll General Practit* 1986;**36**:102–4.
21. Baker R, Streatfield J. What type of general practice do patients prefer? Exploration of practice characteristics influencing patient satisfaction. *Br J Gen Pract* 1995;**45**:654–9.

Management of depression in primary care

ANDRE TYLEE

Michael Shepherd described how the family doctor, as a personal physician, has direct access to the medical history and social background of his patient so that his assessment is influenced by contact with the patient often over many years.[1] In his opening address the President of the Royal College of General Practitioners, Professor Sir Denis Pereira Gray rightly emphasises the importance of continuity of care.

Epidemiology

The National Morbidity Survey indicated that in any week 16% of the United Kingdom population, aged between 16 and 64, suffers from a neurotic disorder, consisting of mixed anxious depression (7.7%), various anxiety states (5%), pure depressive episodes (2.1%), and obsessive–compulsive disorder (1.2%).[2] At least 95% of the population is registered with a general practitioner and over 60% will consult each year. Regarding the older age group, a prevalence rate of between 11% and 16% for depression amongst those over 65 at home in the United Kingdom have been described.[3,4]

Shepherd and colleagues[1] reported that 14% of those registered with their general practitioner would consult for a psychiatric condition in any year. Strathdee and Jenkins[5] estimate that in a practice list of 2000, there would be 60–100 patients with depression, 70–80 with anxiety and 50–60 with a situational disturbance.

Studies of consecutive attendees

WHO collaborative study[6] found that 26% of attendees had at least one psychiatric disorder, according to ICD-10 criteria. The estimated prevalence of these diagnoses was current depression 16.9%, neurasthenia 9.7% and generalised anxiety disorder 7.1%.

Twenty-three per cent of children consecutive attendees (between 7 and 12 years) were diagnosed with psychiatric morbidity consisting, in approximately equal parts, of emotional, conduct or mixed disorders.[7] One-third of adolescents had a psychiatric disorder and most children and adolescents present with somatic symptoms so that their concurrent psychiatric disorders go missed.

Disability

All patients included in the Manchester arm of the WHO study were assessed for disability. Fifty-five per cent of those with an ICD-10-defined psychiatric disorder were rated as having moderate or severe disability. There was no symptom threshold where disability rapidly increased: instead, disability increased in a linear fashion with the number of symptoms a patient has, and also varied with time as symptoms come and go.[8]

Natural history

Mann et al.[9] reported a one-year follow-up of 100 patients with neurotic disorders and found that 48% still met case criteria after one year. 24% recovered early, 52% had run an intermittent course, while 25% had shown persistent symptoms throughout the follow-up period. Similar one-year figures were reported by Wright and Anderson.[10] An eleven-year outcome of the cohort reported in 1981 found that 51% of those traced still met probable case criteria and, judging by self-report and inspection of general practitioner case notes, had suffered continuous psychiatric symptoms for the whole eleven-year follow-up.[11]

The primary care version of ICD-10 (ICD10-PHC)

The ICD10-PHC classification of mental disorders in primary care sets 24 conditions that roughly correspond to those in ICD-10. Each condition is listed by diagnosis (the way in which patients with the condition present to general practitioners; diagnostic features and differential diagnoses) and management (information for the patient and the family; counselling for the patient and the family; medication; and indications for specialist referral).

Designed by psychiatrists and general practitioners, field trials in 19 countries proved reliability. The field trial in England showed that general practitioners expanded their concept of depressive illness, more depressive symptoms were correctly learned, and they increased the number of symptoms required both for a diagnosis of depression, and in order to prescribe antidepressants. More general practitioners as a result advise patients to plan daily activities during their treatment, and on building confidence.[12]

Range of treatments in primary care

Primary care teams need to meet the needs of those with mental health problems who can be appropriately and safely managed without referral to secondary care. Approximately nine out of ten patients with mental health problems are managed entirely in primary care, including a quarter of patients with schizophrenia.[13]

Many of the common mental disorders that can be managed in primary care settings have been the focus of research by psychiatrists, who have set out to transmit their skills to primary care staff in treating these disorders and evaluating the effect. Such researchers demonstrated the ability of general practitioners to assist their patients in primary care settings using behavioural anxiety management techniques,[14] problem-based approaches for major depression, psychotherapy skills,[15] and re-attribution skills in somatisation.[16] Many of these training courses have relied on enthusiastic researcher/trainers providing training to motivated participants willing to be evaluated. Many of these projects have not been replicated to test generalisability to less enthusiastic practices.

The management of depression

Depression is the most common mental disorder in primary care, and responds to both drug and psychological treatments. Both types of treatment produce the same outcome, although psychological treatments may cost more than anti-depressants from the general practitioner.[17] Problem-solving, cognitive behaviour therapy and interpersonal psychotherapy have all been shown to be as effective as antidepressants.[18] There is some evidence that the combination of antidepressants and psychotherapy is most effective – but replication of these findings is needed. The newer antidepressants do not produce better results than the older ones, but side effects are less and therefore patients are more likely to comply with treatment.

The WHO study[6] showed that 45% of ICD-10 depressions were undetected, and of those detected, only about a half received a drug (more likely to be a sedative than an antidepressant). Psychiatrists often express concern about the depressions that are not detected in primary care. In fact these illnesses are (on average) less severe than those detected by general practitioners, and their outcome 12 months later is, if anything, rather better – as would be expected because of their lesser severity at outset. The patients are younger, and less likely to be suicidal at outset. Those detected but not treated with drugs were similar in all respects. Those receiving drugs have the severest illnesses; they are older and more likely to be male. At three months follow up, those treated with antidepressants have fewer symptoms and are less likely to be suicidal than those treated with sedatives – although the two groups were identical at outset. The treatment effect is more marked for the more severe depressions, (with more than nine initial symptoms). At one year, all differences have disappeared.[19]

Psychological therapies and counselling in primary care

In primary care, the entire spectrum of mental health problems is seen, which at the mildest end includes worry, grief, emotional reactions to physical illness or threat of it, or events such as the loss of a job. Many general practitioners have responded to the difficulties of obtaining psychological services for patients by employing on-site counsellors, counselling psychologists, clinical psychologists and psychotherapists. In the early 1990s around a third of practices declared someone who provided 'counselling' in the practice.[20] Generalists also need to use listening skills and within the confines of everyday consultations help their patients formulate problem lists and apply problem-solving as well as help patients cope with insoluble problems. The public prefers to be listened to rather than to receive pills (which a majority consider to be addictive). Public satisfaction with counselling is generally found in primary care randomised controlled trials of counselling, which have been unable to so far demonstrate any benefit over 'treatment as usual' by general practitioners.[21, 22] Such studies also demonstrate satisfaction amongst general practitioners. Resources are finite, and the mental health needs of those with moderate and severe mental illness are often not being met. It is essential that primary care counselling and psychological services adopt more clearly defined care protocols and are properly managed, organised, supervised, monitored and evaluated.

Many attendees in primary care have moderate mental health problems (e.g. depression and anxiety disorders) that could become disabling and chronic if undertreated. Well-proven psychological treatments can be applied by clinical psychologists and well-trained counsellors. Such services, however, vary in availability to primary care suggesting perhaps an enhanced role for primary care nurses. Patients with bipolar disorder and 'treatment resistant' depression are probably best managed mainly by the community mental health services with assistance from primary care.

The role of the primary care nurse

United Kingdom practice nurses are involved often in chronic disease management programmes (e.g. asthma and diabetes) where there is financial reward. They have a key potential role in the management of depression in primary care unless there is a dramatic increase in the numbers of community psychiatric nurses or psychologists. Practice nurses also increasingly collaborate with other primary care nurses (community nurses, health visitors, nurse practitioners, midwives, community psychiatric nurses, etc.) in integrated nursing teams in the United Kingdom. Practice nurses have been successfully trained in the assessment and management of depression,[23] and to use problem-solving in major depression. Health visitors trained in counselling have been shown to benefit women with postnatal depression.

Improving mental health skills of the primary care team

About half of United Kingdom general practitioner trainees do a six-month psychiatry hospital attachment, many of which are considered to be unhelpful for a future generalist career. Few general practitioners have higher professional training in mental health. Most general practitioner training is didactic and unsuitable for learning interviewing or therapy skills.[24, 25] Around a third of general practitioners in England & Wales had undertaken mental health training in the previous three years. Respondents rated their competence in a range of mental health skills as generally average but concerning depression recognition rated themselves average or above average. Nearly two-thirds rated themselves below average at 'counselling' and just over half rated themselves below average using cognitive techniques. Respondents wanted further training in: counselling (25%), stress management (20.8%), cognitive techniques (15%) and assessment of suicide risk (7.5%).

General practitioners in South London[26] preferred small group work and wanted mainly mental health skills training. Depression training changed the behaviour of 18 general practitioners in Gotland[27] and improved patient outcome, although three years later educational effect faded when half of the general practitioners had left Gotland.[28] A recent attempt at replication in Hampshire failed to deliver improvements in recognition or patient outcome.[29] An educational intervention in Germany for general practitioners about anxiety disorders, over two seminars with a mixture of didactic input, case discussion, role-play, use of computers and distance learning materials, showed increased recognition, improved attitudes, changes in referrals and more patients treated in primary care.

Reviewing actual consultations changed behaviour in primary care residents in Charleston, USA. Problem-based interviewing learned in a group setting improved the accuracy of general practitioner trainees as well as experienced general practitioners in assessing emotional distress and these changes persist. General practitioner trainers can transmit these skills to trainees. This approach uses real consultations presented in a facilitated group with the opportunity for skill rehearsal. An alternative method is to use prepared videos in which actors and general practitioners demonstrate microskills, which allow skill rehearsal. Videos have been produced in a variety of subjects such as somatisation disorder, alcohol problems, counselling in depression, dementia, psychosis, anxiety and chronic fatigue. Funding is needed to evaluate many of these packages, which are more time consuming and trainer intensive than programmes like the Gotland or Hampshire project described above. Most continuing medical education (CME) for United Kingdom general practitioners is arranged by district-based general practitioner CME tutors and didactic, hence cheaper, in terms of direct cost.

A previous Chief Medical Officer of England & Wales recommended that the profession should improve the educational process through a Practice Professional Development Plan (PPDP), based on service development plans of the practice, local and national objectives and identified educational need. Plans should be practice-based and use novel forms of learning and run parallel to exisiting educational structures.

A flexible learner-centred approach to continuing professional development has long been advocated, although some general practitioners remain unconvinced. Approaches need to include systematic reading, reflection and audit with formal education being complementary and relevant. A modular approach to CME has been advocated whereby learners, with the help of educational mentors, build up portfolios of review diaries and commentaries on read material and undertake performance review. No formal tradition of mentorship currently exists but there are some signs that the PPDP recommendations are to be funded by the Treasury.

The new primary care groups and primary care trusts in the United Kingdom need greater skills in population needs assessment, care management and quality assurance in all areas. Practice-based training is best as it focuses training on everyday problems and related issues around teamwork, communication and practice management. Multiprofessional audit, the development of practice guidelines and protocols and their implementation, the use of screening instruments and the use of paper-based or computer-aided prompts are needed. Practice teams often require facilitation and mentorship with these approaches.

The Royal College of General Practitioners Unit for Mental Health Education in Primary Care at the Institute of Psychiatry teaches trainers to provide 'whole practice' mental health skills training tailored to educational need. Trainers are mainly general practitioners, nurses or counsellors who work in pairs with practices to elicit whole-practice learning need and to then provide or arrange wanted skills training. A new national network of more than a hundred multiprofessional tutors is therefore developing in parallel to existing educational arrangements funded by primary care groups (PCGs), health authorities, educational consortia and health regions. Research and development funding needs to evaluate the worth of this grassroots, innovative educational endeavour.

References

1. Shepherd M, Cooper M, Brown AC, Katon G, eds. *Psychiatric Illness in General Practice*, Oxford: Oxford University Press, 1966.
2. HMSO (Psychiatric Morbidity) 1995.
3. Livingston G, Hawkins A, Graham N *et al*. The Gospel Oak Study: prevalence rates of dementia, depression and activity limitation among elderly residents in inner London. *Psychol Med* 1990;**20**,(1):137–46.
4. Copeland JRM, Davidson IA, Dewey ME *et al*. Alzheimer's disease, other dementias, depression and pseudodementia: prevalence, incidence and three-year outcome in Liverpool. *Br J Psychiatry*, 1992;**161**:230–9.
5. Strathdee G, Jenkins R. Purchasing mental health care for primary care. In: Thornicroft, G, Strathdee, G, eds. *Commissioning Mental Health Services*, pp.77–83. London: HMSO, 1996.
6. Üstün TB, Sartorius N. *Mental Illness in General Health*. Chichester: John Wiley, 1995.
7. Garralda ME Bailey D. Children with psychiatric disorders in primary care. *J Child Psychol Psychiatry*, 1986;**27**:611–24.
8. Ormel J, Von Korff M, Van den Brink W *et al*. Depression, anxiety and social disability show synchrony of change. *Am J Public Health*, 1993;**83**:385–90.
9. Mann AH, Jenkins R Belsey E. The twelve-month outcome of patients with neurotic illness in general practice. *Psychol Med* 1981;**11**:535–50.
10. Wright AF, Anderson AJB Newly identified psychiatric illness in one general practice: 12-month outcome and the influence of patients' personality. *Br J Gen Pract*, 1995;**45**:83–7.
11. Lloyd KR, Jenkins R, Mann, A. Long-term outcome of patients with neurotic illness in general practice. *BMJ*, 1996;**313**:26–8.
12. Goldberg DP, Sharp D, Nanayakkara K. The field trial of the mental disorders section of ICD-10 designed for primary care. *Family Pract*, 1995;**12**:466–73.
13. Melzer D, Hale A, Malik S *et al*. Community care for patients with schizophrenia one year after hospital discharge. *BMJ*, 1991;**303**:1023–26.
14. Catalan J, Gath D, Edmonds G. The effects of non-prescribing of anxiolytics in general practice: 1. Controlled evaluation of psychiatric and social outcome. *Br J Psychiatry*, 1984;**144**:593–602.
15. Andrews G, Brodaty H. General practitioner as psychotherapist. *Med J Australia*, 1980;**2**:655–59.
16. Gask L, Goldberg DP, Porter R, Creed F. The treatment of somatisation: evaluation of a treatment package with general practice trainees. *J Psychosomatic Res*, 1989;**33**:697–703.
17. Scott A, Freeman C. Edinburgh primary care depression study. *BMJ*, 1991;**304**:883–87.
18. Schulberg HC, Block MR, Madonia MJ *et al*. Treating major depression in primary care practice. Eight month clinical outcomes. *Arch Gen Psychiatry*, 1996;**53**:913–9.
19. Goldberg DP, Privett M, Üstün B *et al*. The effects of detection and treatment on the outcome of major depression in primary care: a naturalistic study in 15 cities. *Br J Gen Pract* (in press).
20. Sibbald B, Addington-Hall J, Brenneman D, Freeling P. Counsellors in English and Welsh general practices; their nature and distribution. *BMJ*. 1993;**306**:29–33.
21. Harvey L, Nelson SJ, Lyons RA *et al*. A randomised controlled trial and economic evaluation of counselling in primary care. *Br J Gen Pract*, 1998; **48**:1043–8.
22. Friedli K, King MB, Lloyd M, Horder J. Randomised controlled assessment of non-directive psychotherapy versus routine general practitioner care. *Lancet*, 1997;**350**:1662–5.
23. Wilkinson G. The role of the practice nurse in the management of depression. *Int Rev Psychiatry*, 1992;**4**:311–6.

24. Turton P, Tylee A, Kerry S. Mental health training needs in general practice. *Primary Care Psychiatry*, 1995;**1**:197–9.
25. Singleton A, Tylee A. Continuing medical education in mental illness: a paradox for general practitioners. *Br J Gen Pract*, 1996;**46**:339–41.
26. Kerwick S, Jones R, Mann A *et al.* Mental healthcare training priorities in general practice. *Br J Gen Pract*, 1997;**47**:225–7.
27. Rutz W, Von Knorring, L, Walinker J *et al.* Effect of an educational program for general practitioners on Gotland on the pattern of prescription of psychotropic drugs. *Acta Psychiatr Scand*, 1990;**82**:399–403.
28. Rutz W, Von Knorring L, Walinder J. Long-term effects of an educational program for general practitioners given by the Swedish Committee for the Prevention and Treatment of Depression. *Acta Psychiatr Scand*, 1992;**85**:83–8.
29. Thompson C, Kinmonth AL, Stevens L *et al.* Effects of a clinical-practice guideline and practice-based education on detection and outcome of depression in primary care: Hampshire Depression Project randomised controlled trial. *Lancet*, 2000;**355**:185–91.

National Service Framework for Mental Health

ANDRE TYLEE and ANN DAWSON

This is a brief overview of the National Framework for Mental Health, (NSF), which focuses on mental health needs of adults up to 65 years of age. While the NSF touches on the needs of children and young people, these are being addressed more fully through a separate service development programme across the NHS and social services. An NSF for older people to be published in the spring of 2000 will include mental health needs.

At any one time, one adult in six suffers from one or other form of mental illness, in other words, mental illnesses are as common as asthma. They range from more common conditions, such as depression, to schizophrenia, which affects fewer than one person in a hundred. Mental illness is not well understood; it frightens people and all too often it carries a stigma.

Most people with mental health problems are cared for by their general practitioners within a primary care team (PCT) and this is what they

Editorial note:

In *The New NHS* the United Kingdom Government stated that it was its intention to work with the profession and representatives of users and carers to establish clearer, evidence-based National Service Frameworks (NSFs) for major areas and disease groups, to ensure that nationally patients get greater consistency in the availability and quality of services. NSFs will set standards and define service models for a defined service of care group, put in place strategies to support implementation, establish performance measures against which progress within an agreed time scale will be measured, and provide advice. The first NSF to be developed was in the field of mental health.

Grateful thanks are given to the Department of Health for permission to reprint sections of the NSF for Mental Health in the following text and to PriMHE.

prefer. Generally, for every hundred individuals who consult their general practitioner with a mental health problem, nine will be referred to a specialist service for assessment, and advice/treatment.

Some people with severe mental illness require care from specialist services working in partnership with the independent sector and other agencies that would provide housing, training and employment.

National Service Framework standards

NSF has set standards in seven areas. Each standard is based on the evidence and knowledge base available and supported by service models of examples of good practice. The standards are listed below.

1 Health and social services should:
- promote mental health for all working with individuals and communities;
- combat discrimination against individuals and groups with mental health problems, and promote social inclusions.

2 Any service user who contacts a primary health care team with a common mental health problem should:
- have their mental health needs identified and assessed;
- be offered effective treatments, including referral to a specialist for further assessment, treatment and care if they require it.

3 Any individual with a mental health problem should:
- be able to make contact around the clock with the local services to meet their needs and receive adequate care;
- be able to use NHS Direct as it develops for first-level advice and referral on to a specialist help lines or local services.

4 All mental health service users under the Care Programme Approach (CPA), should:
- receive care which optimises engagement, prevents or anticipates crisis and reduces risk;
- have a copy of a written care plan which:
  - includes the action to be taken in a crisis by service users, their carers and their care co-ordinator;
  - advises general practitioners how they should respond if the service user needs additional help;
  - is regularly reviewed by their care co-ordinator;
- enables them to access service 24 hours a day, 365 days a year.

5 Each service user who is assessed as requiring a period of care away from their homes should have:
- timely access to an appropriate hostel bed or alternative place which is:

    – in the least constrictive environment with the need to protect them and the public;

    – as close to home as possible;

- a copy of a written care plan agreed on discharge which sets out the care to be provided, identifies the care co-ordinator and specifies the action to be taken in a crisis.

6 All individuals who provide regular and substantial care for a person on CPA should:

- have an assessment of their care in physical and mental needs repeated on at least an annual basis;
- have their own written care plan, which is given to them and implemented in discussion with them.

7 Local health and social care communities should prevent suicides by:

- promoting mental health for all, working with individuals and communities (standard one);
- delivering high quality primary mental health care (standard two);
- ensuring that anyone with a mental health problem can contact local services via the primary care team, a helpline or an accident and emergency Department (standard three);
- ensuring that the individuals with severe and enduring mental illness have a care plan which meets their specific needs including access to services round the clock (standard four);
- providing safe hospital accommodation for individuals who need it (standard five);
- enabling individuals caring for someone with severe mental illness to receive the support which they need to continue to care (standard six).

and in addition:

- supporting local prison staff in preventing suicides among prisoners;
- ensuring that staff are competent to assess the risk of suicide among individuals at greatest risk;
- developing local systems for suicide audit to learn lessons and take any necessary action.

Making it happen

Implementing the NSF will require new patterns of local partnerships and team work, with mental health assuming priority for the NHS and social care organisations, and their partners. To secure and sustain change, strong leadership and clear commitment from clinician managers, combined with effective engagement with all who have responsibility for improving mental health services, will be essential. For the first time, change in mental health is being fostered and directed with a clear expectation of what should be achieved. Firm and supportive performance management at local, regional and national level will further ensure that capacity and capability are maximised and positive change encouraged and valued. No one should underestimate the enormity of the task for a much needed strategy to raise the mental wealth of the nation. Organisations such as PriMHE, a UK national association specialising in primary care mental health education, are totally committed to helping with implementation of the NSF.

Treatment of depression in a managed care setting

PETER JUHN

At the outset let me make a few disclaimers: firstly, I am not a psychiatrist; secondly, I am not a scientist and thirdly, I am not really an expert either! But what I am is something that you might not have ever heard about. I am a 'health delivery systems engineer'. What we do is look at health delivery to see if the insights we have gained from science can be applied to the design of healthcare systems.

There are three things I want to cover. Firstly, to give you a sense of the Kaiser Permanente system and also the Care Management Institute and what we do at Kaiser. Secondly, to describe the care management approach that we have developed for depression. This is very much an engineering approach based on the science that several of the previous speakers have talked about. The third is to share with you some of the data that we have been collecting that begins to describe the processes of care.

Kaiser Permanente

To begin with Kaiser Permanente: it is a very large – in fact it is probably the largest – private, non-profit healthcare delivery organisation worldwide. We provide comprehensive 'cradle to grave' coverage for nearly nine million members in the United States. We are the pioneer of the prepaid group practice form of managed care, commonly known as HMO or Health Maintenance Organisation. Our aspiration is not unlike your aspiration, which is really to be a world leader in improving health through affordable and integrated healthcare. Looking at the map of the Kaiser Permanente organisation, there are 16 states in which we are represented, we have almost nine million members and there are 10000 physicians that work exclusively

97

within Kaiser Permanente. There are another 75 000 non-physicians; included in this group are about 30 000 nurses and pharmacists. There are about 8000 hospital beds in our system, about 300 medical offices and 30 medical centres. It is a very large organisation, with a revenue base of over $15 billion dollars annually.

The Care Management Institute

Within Kaiser there is the Care Management Institute, which I direct. We are trying to focus delivery around knowledge-based decisions, member-centred outcomes and technology tools. We really want to help our patients achieve optimum health. The definition we use for care management is co-ordinated healthcare for logical groupings of patients, including patients with depression. Looking at this prospectively, to improve, maintain, or limit the degradation of their optional status – this is not about waiting until someone gets sick and then intervening, it is about looking at the prospective ways of treating patients.

CMI, or Care Management Institute, also stands for:

- content;
- measurement; and
- implementation

because those are the three activities that we are engaged in. Professor Kleinman mentioned that our organisation is a research organisation; it is really research with a small 'r'. It is more of an 'r' and 'd' organisation; the 'd' part is really the development of the engineered approaches and also the deployment of all the programmes throughout Kaiser Permanente.

We have been focusing on eight programme areas of which depression is one of the key ones. We have not covered all of the conditions; we have deliberately chosen those with high morbidity. There is also ample evidence in the literature that many of you have produced that actually suggests there are better ways of treatment. The measurement aspect of our work is looking at specific outcomes for the various priority areas. The most important thing that we do is implementation: in my organisation there are about 70 people who are actually focused on the implementation side, because this is really where 'the rubber meets the road'. This is where we take those concepts and actually get them applied to our members.

Some background facts may be known to some of you here but nevertheless bear repeating and are as follows.

- Thirty per cent of patients in primary care come in depressed, whether they know it, or whether the provider knows it.
- Six per cent of the US population will, at some point in their history, develop depression.
- Depression is twice as common in women.

This type of information is very important for an organisation like ours, because we have a set premium that comes in and with those premiums ($15.6 billion in revenue) we need to make sure that we can provide adequately for all the nine million people who are getting care through Kaiser. They are very high utilisers of healthcare.

There are significant numbers of people at work who are depressed. Being depressed at work gives you increased absenteeism and reduced productivity from an employer perspective. The total estimated cost of absenteeism in the United States is about $44 billion. This is just looking at short-term disability: depressive disorders really count significantly higher than many other disability-causing conditions. Looking at short-term disability among mental health diagnoses, depressive disorders account for more than half.

Kaiser's depression programme

Let me tell you a little bit about our depression programme, what it is and how it was developed. It is a primary care-based programme, meaning it really has in its sights the care our primary care providers – whether they are physicians, nurses, nurse practitioners – are actually providing on a daily basis to our members. I should also mention that on a weekly basis Kaiser Permanente has about 100 000 patient encounters. It is based on clinical practice guidelines, which are in turn based on evidence – evidence that has been found in the scientific literature. Where there is a shortage of evidence, it means using our own internal experts within psychiatry to help us resolve those areas.

It is also based on case identification, the whole notion of 'you cannot improve unless you manage' and 'you can't manage unless you measure', which is predicated on having information systems that allow us to do that. Physician education is also a very important component. Patient education is important because we want to encourage patients to be partners in their treatment and follow the various approaches to care. It is very important that treatment co-ordination is a key notion, bringing in the various parties who need to be working together as a team and in that team a very essential player is the patient. The mental health specialist, psychiatrist and others need to be involved, but it is not really the starting point because in our system, much like the National Health Service (NHS), a lot of the initial diagnosis needs to come through the primary care provider.

Physician pocket card

A practical thing we have developed is the 'physician pocket card'. We have made these available to our physicians – it is a laminated card that they can stick in their white coat or can keep on their desktop when they are seeing patients. The first pocket card was on diagnosis, the second is on treatment. This is not very sophisticated in the sense that a lot of science has not gone into it. It is basic enough that it can be quickly looked at and quickly give the tips that are needed to treat the patients.

Algorithm of care

There is also the algorithm of care. Our guidelines look at risk factors and diagnostic criteria and then the various facets of treatment, the recommended medications, as well as special populations. It is a series of questions and then a kind of branching logic from those questions. We also have tools that are focused on the patient – some of these are pamphlets: simple, straightforward things just describing what depression is, what self-help techniques there might be, even a symptoms quiz. The latter is not as sophisticated as a health status questionnaire, but again it is something that can be done very readily. It can even give you, at a crude level, a way of identifying these patients. Also it tries to get into the engaging of patients into a partnership, letting them know about different treatment choices and helping find what treatment choices can work best for them, in this case, antidepressants, counselling, combined therapy. Then there is also information about medications, what side effects to look out for, how to deal with these side effects, when to come and when to be seen by a provider.

Results of process-based outcome studies

I would now like to discuss the outcome studies we have been doing. These are not looking to see whether patients are better or worse, these are really process of care outcomes, service delivery process outcomes. We have looked at our population and have a database of about 320 000 patients who are being followed. We looked at the prevalence of depression, visits to the mental health provider, use of antidepressants, a depression diagnosis or support diagnosis among those receiving medication and then various antidepression measures. We also looked at the three most common types of depressive illness: major depression, Dysthymia and subthreshold conditions and then we looked at a number of these issues to see whether or not the patient would be included in the study. It is very important for us that this kind of study is rigorous and has credibility with the providers. So we have been looking at a study population of about 3.5 million members. About 320 000 patients were identified within those numbers in a cross-sectional observation during one year, 1998.

We found that about 5% of our membership receives a depression diagnosis – that is more than our heart disease population, diabetes population or asthma population. Much of the care of the depressed patients occurs entirely within primary care, so we do not do a lot of referral to specialist care. About 50% of the patients are diagnosed by a primary care practitioner; less than 20% of those diagnosed are actually referred on to a mental health specialist.

Antidepressant therapy is frequently used to treat depression, but it is also used to treat conditions other than depression. About 10% of the adults in our entire population, almost 900 000 people, received some type of antidepressant therapy in 1998. Fifteen per cent of this was actually prescribed not in the category of depression (the three categories I told you about earlier).

There are certain guidelines of care published by the Agency of Healthcare Policy and Research. One of the subguidelines within the depression guidelines refers to the duration of therapy and the frequency of follow-up visits. What we found is that only 15% of the patients in our system are actually getting the required duration of care. Depression in females is twice as high as in men. Looking at the role of primary care and mental health specialists, psychiatrists, psychologists, in diagnosing new episodes of depression, you see that it is virtually the same overall. But there are various systems of care, various regions that we have operations in, where there are significant variations – for instance, most of the diagnosis is done in primary care (almost 80%) in one region whereas in another region it can be the reverse.

Looking at antidepressant use among age groups, again in our various systems of care there is variation from system to system in how much antidepressant use there is, but also within one of these systems there is variation with the various age categories as well. As to what type of medications are being used, most of the first-line therapy is selective serotonin-reuptake inhibitor (SSRI) treatment with a much smaller amount of tricyclic antidepressant (TCA) use. We looked at the clinical indication of how many of the people being treated with antidepressants are actually depressed or have other supporting diagnoses of depression and then how many of these are unknown clinical indications. There is a substantial number – 20% – that really do not have a known clinical indication.

Let me just conclude by saying that depression is a very significant problem for Kaiser Permanente and it is something that we recognise. We are investing in it to learn more about it and also to develop very practical tools that actually treat our depressed patients. Our process–outcome study, looking at 300 000 patients, pinpoints significant opportunities for us to improve care through provider education and changes to our system. Then the depression care management programme must focus on providing tools again. The way we can deploy these technologies, deploy the tools, is by using our website. The website right now has about 20 000 visits a day, so there is a significant amount of activity. Through this website we have both on-line CMI education on depression and also all of the programmes that I described for you about depression. I should also mention that for those of you who are interested, we make available all of our guidelines to the public. The website address is pkc.kp.org.

To finish, there are major opportunities for us to improve depression care. We are basing a lot of what we do on the evidence that is being produced by the scientists in this room. But we really need to start moving beyond learning more and start taking what we know to make some tools, apply those tools and then see whether their application leads to population improvement.

Depression – a patient's view of the future

RICHARD HORNSBY

Last night while I was talking to Arthur Kleinman and in a rash moment said that I feel a little bit, and sometimes a large bit, like an outsider – for I am not a medical professional of any sort. Arthur, in his own words, was quick 'to cut to the chase' and told me that I had it *all wrong* and that I was perhaps *the only true insider*, as I have lived with this very difficult illness for many years, and it forms the basis and theme of my talk.

Contrary to public opinion and some professional opinion, depression is a life-threatening illness. In my experience it is seldom treated as such. I am asked to speak on behalf of patients or sufferers from depression, and this is an onerous responsibility. One thing I know is that anyone who has not suffered from depression has little knowledge of what this illness is and how it affects the individual. I am only too aware that many people get poorly diagnosed and poorly treated. I am aware of the horrible and often terrifying journey that people with depression undertake often alone and often without adequate information. My concern has been to provide some reliable guidelines so that people can find their way through their illness and back into a productive life. Depression is either not understood at all by friends and family or it is grossly oversimplified. There is much evidence to suggest that depression is a chronic ongoing illness for many sufferers and one that requires constant monitoring, treatment and drug therapy. There is also a facile notion that if you simply swallow the pills, it will all miraculously disappear.

I must take issue with the statements made at this meeting that general practitioners have the time, or are expert in diagnosing and treating depression. In the same way as patients should be screened for other diseases I propose that it is the right of anyone suffering from depression –

or thought to be – to have at least one consultation with a psychiatrist. This would be a great step forward. And I should remind the audience that the Prime Minister, Tony Blair, observed in the letter he sent to me 'we [must] tackle the underlying social, economic and environmental conditions as well as the specific causes'. As an organiser and as a patient I have asked myself what would actually make this a successful meeting – and I think the pertinent answer must be if it acts as a beginning of a real change in the way society perceives and deals with depressive illness.

It was William Styron who moved mountains in the understanding of clinical depression when he wrote *Darkness Visible*, the account of his experience of this illness. In it he wrote:

> What I began to discover is that, mysteriously and in ways that are totally remote from normal experience, the grey drizzle of horror induced by depression takes on the quality of physical pain ... there is no escape from this smothering confinement, it is entirely natural that the victim begins to think ceaselessly of oblivion.

What surprised him, and made this work a bestseller, was that by articulating the experience of depression he had spoken to millions of people who had not been able to adequately describe their own struggle with depression. Illnesses of the mind need those who suffer them to document them, in order to make intelligible what otherwise seems unknowable to those lucky enough to escape this awful illness – those who think that depression is the experience of a bunch of malingerers who cannot cope with life.

I do not want to list the litany of woes that an individual experiences, but as I elected to speak as a patient I must set out something of the workings out of this illness, both in myself and in my family. I lost my father to this illness, our home, my own depressions have cost me my health for many years, my ability to work and get through financial difficulties, and eventually destroyed my marriage. Even today I admit to times when I feel fated by genes, fated by the feeling of having been dealt the wrong hand of cards to cope at times with a life that has often seemed overwhelmingly difficult. As Edgar Allan Poe once succinctly put the genetic twist when writing of a character afflicted by moods and madness: 'It was, he said, constitutional and a family evil, and one for which he despaired to find a remedy.'

It is now over twenty years since my father killed himself, a victim of his depression and increasing uncontrollable moods. As many others, I know how suicide cuts through your life like nothing else; leaving one left trying to make sense of the insensible. Suicide leaves a terrible trail of devastation like a tornado that rips through the heartland of spouses, relatives and uncomprehending friends. It is dreadful in its effects upon the living. It becomes, as Alvarez wrote in *The Savage God*, a condition that is 'airless and without exits'. No one who has suffered from depression could equate it with unhappiness; the nearest normal human response to depression is to be found in the loss of grieving and bereavement. Although I am far from being a signed up Freudian, this sense of loss was movingly described by Sigmund Freud, who wrote to his friend Ludwig Binswanger after the death of his friend's son:

> We find a place for what we lose. Although we know that after such a loss the acute stage of mourning will subside, we also know that we shall remain inconsolable and will never find a substitute. No matter what may fill the gap, even if it be filled completely, it nevertheless remains something else.

Over a period of time I have come to believe more and more that mental health is one of the crucial underpinning concepts and conditions that make for a civilised society. While we know that animals can exhibit some of the physical manifestations of depression, it seems that only in our species are we able to reflect on our own condition and also try and regulate its dysfunction. I am also increasingly convinced that depression and mood disorders are a broad church. In a great many cases depression seems to strike families and it is not a complicated matter to trace its genetic lineage. In society today there is an additional component that is driving depression and it is a common cause – increased and increasing levels of stress.

People today have to put up with adaptations in work, and in family life, all of which put enormous strains on their emotional as well as physical resources. All too often this adaptation is not able to be processed, and people are left feeling as if they are out of control of their world and their environment. Seligman was one of the first to point out that hopelessness and inability to have control over one's life is also a key precipitator of depression. The wide remit of this meeting has looked not simply at the genetic components of depression, or purely at depressives as individuals with a medical condition. Under the benign influence of Arthur Kleinman's broad-ranging perspective, it has drawn upon all the social and societal influences that have precipitated a global crisis in mental healthcare – and particularly in the treatment of depression and anxiety disorders.

It is strange to think that as we are about to launch into the new millennium that it is estimated that last year over 30 000 Americans committed suicide.

- More people die from suicide than from homicide in the United States.
- In the United States on an average day, 84 people die from suicide and an estimated 1900 adults attempt suicide.
- In the United Kingdom and Ireland there were 6426 suicides.
- Seventy-five per cent of successful suicides are by males.

- Suicide is the second leading cause of death in young people.
- The rising trend of suicide shows a 50% increase since 1990.

These chilling figures do not seem to be cause for great celebration.

My memories of my father linger on in a sad unfinished epitaph to an interrupted and largely wasted life, and my own depressions later made me feel as if I was walking in his footsteps to the edge of a perilous abyss. And in all this, it has brought home to me that after the 'Decade of the Brain' the public by and large is ignorant, frightened, and still stigmatises those with mental illness. This manifests in all sorts of differing ways as we have heard. But, in our wisdom, since the 1960s we have closed our institutions, we have sent those with profound despair and inability to cope into lonely rooms in which they can eke out an existence with a quality of life that is perhaps less than zero. There is no longer any asylum for those in need, in the true and proper sense of the word.

Where one might ask in this civilised developed country are the 24-hour walk-in help centres to help the desperate and suicidal? Where can those with depression go and receive care when their families can no longer cope? Where are the signs of a mental health infrastructure that really works for patients and takes account of their needs?

Depressives are an easy group to push aside because they do not make too much fuss. They also carry a burden of guilt as they can see the suffering that their illness also causes to others. However they need to try and be more vocal and especially in reaction to prejudice. In the meantime there are many caring charities and voluntary organisations at work to help those with depression, who try to fill the gap created by overwhelming indifference.

Part of society's response to depression must in my opinion also be a push for better and more effective treatments. Having spoken about the social dimension of depression, I would also like to stand resolutely behind my commitment to pharmacological treatment of this illness. I honestly believe that if it were not for the fact that I am 'still taking the pills' that I would not be standing in front of you today. My depression was so overwhelming that self-destruction did not seem selfish and cruel but the only logical and reasonable way to stop the pain of the present. I do not believe that anybody who commits suicide really wants to end their own life at all. What they want to find is some way, any way, to escape the all-consuming present that has become unendurable.

If someone were to ask me as a patient what I would like to see in the future, I would first look towards new and better drug therapies, as we understand more about the human brain. Although the newer generation of antidepressants are a considerable advancement on older-generation drugs, they still do not represent the quantum leap that I feel is called for. We need drugs that lift people out of depression in days not weeks, and we need drugs without side effects, and we need drugs that actually cure depression. I am grateful to Professor Berndt for his remarks that show the gap between what antidepressants should deliver and the present state of science – when up to 50% of patients in the real world do not respond adequately, and a considerable number do not respond at all. We still need intensive research into the biology of depression. But all this cannot be at the expense of rational demands placed upon individuals and society as a whole. Depression is, as we have learned, not simply a condition to be cured by swallowing pills for a few weeks. It also has deep and profound roots in society. As a patient I believe that there must be a proper commitment to the practice of psychiatry or it will become totally marginalised – and I believe that that is unacceptable – and I also urge psychiatry to listen to the voices of those whom it is dedicated to serve. I also urge general practitioners to be better trained in treating depression, and better listeners to the narratives of their patients.

It was Professor Simon Wessely who pointed out the complexities of somatisation in depression. These interwoven personal narratives cannot be disentangled and assessed in a visit of no more than four minutes. I think that the only way this will be corrected is if we, as patient advocacy groups and professionals, join together and under a common consensus demand the right to the speciality care that this illness should command. And as well as demanding higher standards of treatment, we, as patients, must actively support the profession from which we expect support – namely psychiatry.

Today, psychiatrists seem to be treated only as wardens for the acutely mentally ill; they have no time or position within our health system to devote to the much larger problem of depression. They seem to have become dislocated from the very group that their profession was expected to serve. In any talk of setting agendas for better quality care in the next millennium, we are faced with some profound and difficult questions about how we should act towards one another, and what is acceptable to a civilised society. These questions are universal, and like human rights they apply across the entire world – in the developed and the developing worlds. We now have some indication of the scale of the problem, and we also know a considerable amount about possible solutions. At least we can see the way ahead. A great deal has been spelled out to us here at this meeting that could have enormous impact. The real test of commitment however will be if these solutions can be turned into practical realities, and if they cannot then I fear for us all, and for patients in particular.

The worst outcome for between 15% and 30% of severe depressive cases is suicide, and as Kay Redfield Jamison points out in her new and compelling study of suicide, *Night Falls Fast*:

It is a societal illusion that suicide is rare. It is not. Certainly the mental illnesses most closely tied to suicide are not rare. They are common conditions, and unlike cancer and heart disease, they disproportionately affect and kill the young

I suggest that if we care about all our futures these are issues that can no longer be avoided.

But there are two crucial points I must further address – what do we mean by the 'successful treatment of depression'? And to this pivotal notion I must mention the helpful conversations I have had with Alex Cohen of the World Mental Health Project, whose insights clarified the need to make this clear. Do we mean, as the media would have us believe some sort Huxleyian Brave New World – 'Soma' pills to end all our human sufferings? If this is anyone's idea of what the outcome of depression should be, or is, then I suggest we need to think the whole thing through again. This sort of media hype is demeaning to depression and its reality.

In my view, and I hope others will agree, the proper outcome of treating depression is not happiness – happiness is only a fortunate component of a life. The successful outcome of treating depression is giving people back emotional literacy, so that they can engage in the day-to-day realities of life – even to experience profound sadness and suffering in a way that has meaning. It is giving people back the ability to act with reason, and not to be trapped and dragged down in the 'grey drizzle' that Styron so accurately characterised.

And the last thing is this – that it has become abundantly clear, both through my own experiences and driven home by this meeting, that the greatest stumbling block to making any real difference in the treatment of depression and other related mental disorders is stigma. Stigma is the real barrier to better care. No one body or organisation will ever achieve what is needed to break down the walls of ignorance and stigma. I therefore thought what our charity's most appropriate response to this meeting should be. I have therefore proposed an International Collaboration for the Prevention of Stigma in Mental Illness, which I hope organisations across the world will sign up for. This will be a large undertaking and it will require goodwill from many diverse parties. But I sense that if we do not pull together all the organisations worldwide who work in this field – advocacy groups, mental health professionals and ordinary people (since we all know someone with this illness) – then there will be lots of rumbling, talk, interesting meetings such as this but in the end nothing will change. Anyone interested in following these developments should look at our websites www.stigma.org and www.depression.org.uk.

I think I speak for everyone here when I say I am appalled that people are still afraid of their jobs, their mortgages, and living a normal life if they say they have, or have had, this illness – depression. I am equally sickened by the examples of those who eke out a life, their lives bereft of family, friends and any human dignity, because of an illness that is far from their choosing, and only because of ignorance and prejudice manifesting in the all too familiar guise of stigma. We do not need more depression, or more statistics – we have seen the scale of human suffering. By 2020, if we do nothing, depression will be the second leading cause of death worldwide. We don't need much more talk either – we need only to act on what we know, and on what has been made so very obvious throughout by all the distinguished speakers. I hope that I have been able to adequately express the views and hopes of millions of people who suffer from depression, and who too often have no voice. We all hope that the important messages conveyed here at this conference will grow and flourish into a response to these needs and into action.

Depression and the Workplace

Overview

This next section deals with a very important consequence of depression. Typically out of every hundred employees, twenty will be suffering from depression, more often than not stress induced. Job-related stress has huge consequences for companies of every kind. Bad management, which is the usual reason for this fast and growing problem, can drive a company to the point where 50–60% of the workforce are suffering from depression. In addition up to 25% of absenteeism is due to back pain and 25% of back pain is due to depression. It is worth noting here that in the United Kingdom back pain accounts for 119 million days of certified incapacity, consumes 112 million general practitioner consultations and 800 000 hospital inpatient days.

Psychological hazards are potentially harder to identify than physical hazards in the workplace. Thus it is important that the occupational physician works closely with the employer. There is now growing awareness worldwide, and certainly by the United Kingdom's Health and Safety Commission and Executive, that occupational health problems, including mental health, are priority areas that need addressing urgently.

Health risk management of depression in the United Kingdom workplace

KEVIN HOLLAND-ELLIOTT

Background to risk management in the United Kingdom

The *Implementing Turnbull, A Boardroom Briefing*[1] produced by the Chartered Institute of Accountants, advises how quoted companies should assess their business risk in all areas, and manage it. These risks will include developing new business, controlling investments and managing the cost base of the organisation. Most of those business risks materialise as a result of decision-making. How then can a business afford to overlook the mental health of its workforce? The problem when looking at the cost base is that payroll costs, costs of injury, legal claims, ill health retirement, recruiting replacements and sickness absence will be accounted for in different parts of the organisation, therefore reducing the visibility of the whole. In addition, there is currently no linking of mental health to risk performance. Furthermore, with 'free' National Health Service (NHS) healthcare there is no culture of organisational intervention as a healthcare purchaser in the United Kingdom and no government champion, such as a workers' insurance scheme, to directly fund early and effective rehabilitation or treatment. The same spread of cost applies when employees are dismissed for poor performance or retired early. The NHS, Department of Social Security (DSS), other government departments, private health funds, insurance companies, pension funds and the employer, all share the cost of treatment and social security payments when employees can no longer work. This may be the best way to carry a risk in general, i.e. spread it, but it deprives the employee of a champion. To plagiarise Balint's phrase, 'there is a collusion of anonymity'.

113

Hazard identification, risk assessment and control

Health and Safety law in the United Kingdom is primarily driven by Regulations enacted under the Health and Safety at Work Act etc. 1974. There is growing realisation by the Health and Safety Commission and Executive that occupational health problems, including mental health, are priority issues to address, and they have attempted to communicate this to employers.[2] Current law already places upon employers a duty to identify all relevant hazards and manage the risk. In addition, the Disability Discrimination Act 1995 places a duty of non-discrimination on employers with regard to mentally ill employees if they qualify.[3] Mental health issues arising from and at work are therefore already legislated for. In addition, at Common Law, employees can successfully sue for compensation if negligence can be proven.[4]

Psychological hazards are, in principle, no more difficult to identify than physical hazards such as toxic chemicals. Nurses working on a locked psychiatric ward with potentially violent patients and security-van workers delivering cash are at risk of experiencing trauma. Employees facing major organisational change and uncertainty are 'more at risk' of feeling pressured. However, much 'pressure' originates from sources nothing to do with work. It is the lack of a formal way of assessing the severity of these pressures as felt by individuals that is at the heart of the issue. Even if affected to the point of mental illness, most people continue to come to work, and are then more vulnerable due to their condition. A bullying manager or unsympathetic approach from the organization can tip people in this situation into despair, long-term sickness and even premature retirement. In the worst cases employees develop avoidance behaviour towards their former employer and everything that reminds them of it.

Health risk appraisal tools can be used to map the prevalence of depression using the General Health Questionnaire (GHQ) in one of its forms, or other validated tools. I have presented to some organisations where as many as 60% of employees score as 'cases' of mental ill health, i.e. with a GHQ12 scoring four or more. A more normal level would be 15–20%.[5] This means that even in a 'healthy' organization of 1000 persons, 150–200 would be mentally 'not well', though usually still at work. I have frequently experienced a response rate of ≥80% to health risk questionnaires if supported properly by the organisation; however, employees can be wary of approaches to detecting and measuring depression. Cultural factors are crucial in gaining acceptance, and clear and honest leadership from the board is essential for any initiative to work. Where this is not forthcoming, mental health problems tend to be submerged and may be more prevalent. Personality assessment and management style of the board, linked to the prevalence of mental health problems in an organisation, may be an interesting area for further research.

Modern approaches to risk assessment questionnaires via the Internet or organisational intranet[6] can provide an interactive format for the employee and a good source of links to further advice and support. They can also provide anonymous data that an organisation can use for monitoring and planning health initiatives. The data may show 'hot spots' of mental health problems within an organisation, which should lead to a formal risk assessment. Sickness absence information, employee and customer attitude surveys, insurance claims and turnover of staff can all be used as indicators. By identifying these areas in advance of serious problems, intervention in the form of management improvement can theoretically reduce or eliminate the problem. There is a paucity of quality research in this area.

Using absence management as a process to identify and manage health risk

When an employee becomes a 'case' to the employer, it will be as a result of poor performance, absence or both. There are two absence management processes to manage, long term and short term. Absence of less than 14 days' duration is my working definition for short-term absence. Management of this type of absenteeism should be primarily a line management responsibility, looking for patterns in the organisation's absence or patterns in an individual record. Conditions commonly detected by this approach can include depression, alcohol abuse and other long-term health conditions that, whilst they are usually stable, can be prone to exacerbation. These conditions may be covered by the Disability Discrimination Act 1995 and need fair procedures and skilled advice to be handled properly. Without a good communication link between clinician, occupational physician and employer, future employment can be put in jeopardy. Understanding organisational culture and workplace ergonomic factors are important, as some cases are caused or exacerbated by work. This needs to be managed as part of the overall clinical treatment plan. This is a particular problem in the absence of an occupational physician, when the general practitioner, with no direct knowledge of the specific workplace or its culture, must liaise directly with management. With approximately 500 specialists in occupational medicine practising in the United Kingdom for 28 million workers this is likely to be the normal state of affairs.

As accidents decline in frequency and severity, occupational medical problems are more important for organisations as a source of legal claims. This is a significant risk exposure for most organisations, and good sickness absence monitoring can be the best way to spot problems developing. Bouts of respiratory illnesses amongst paint sprayers must immediately put employers on their guard regarding occupational asthma. Musculoskeletal absence in call centres must put employers on notice for work related upper-limb problems. Depression can also be an important component of physical diseases, especially when prolonged, and it sometimes needs the occupational physician to be a good advocate on behalf of the employee to deal with perceptions of malingering, particularly in association with chronic back pain.

Absence lasting longer than 21 days is usually due to significant physical or psychosocial disease. The diagnosis and whether the condition is caused or made worse by work need to be known by clinicians. Later, when the employee is recovering, good communication with management, the employee, the employee's clinicians and occupational health advisers is needed to rehabilitate the employee. Rehabilitation, resettlement to alternative work, retraining, medical retirement or dismissal on grounds of capability may all need to be considered. Given current employment law and the Disability Discrimination Act 1995 in particular, this is a medico-legal minefield for employers. Skilled human resource and occupational medical advice is therefore essential. In a workplace setting, the key relationship is between the employer and the employee by virtue of the employment contract, and when off sick with depression it is the employee who is in breach of contract. Doctors often fail to appreciate that their patient can be legitimately dismissed when not capable of work. Only good clinical treatment and advocacy on behalf of the patient can prevent this. In my experience, most employers are anxious to do their best for the employee but lack of information nor clinical progress, particularly with regard to vague prognoses, can be decisive in a decision to dismiss when there is pressure on budgets. In the United Kingdom the organisation bears the cost of the absence, but once the employee is dismissed or retired, the costs are transferred to other bodies: insurers, the occupational pension funds or, most commonly, the state.

Ideally, with the employees consent, liaison between the occupational physician and the general practitioner should persuade management to give realistic time for medical management of the case. In the later stages, when the diagnosis and prognosis are known, rehabilitation back to work can be planned. Flexibility from both the management and employee is crucial to rehabilitation success. The occupational physician has a pivotal role in assessing function, and liaising with all the stakeholders including the patient's general practitioner. Most organisations wish to keep experienced personnel and so a good link with the clinician, within ethical guidelines, is in the patient's best interest. Employees with depression may face delays when they need access to secondary care assessment, treatment and support services. Employers sometimes pay for speedier assessment.

Summary

Depression is a common problem affecting approximately one-fifth of workers, most of whom remain at work. The risks to safety or corporate governance from the underlying ≥20% of workers who are not well remains unaccounted for and largely unrecognised. Poor visibility of the scale and cost of the problem, together with inadequate cost-benefit analysis mean that the will or expertise to actively manage depression in the workplace is not present, as it is simpler and cheaper to dismiss or retire depressed employees when they become too much of a problem. A business case remains to be developed on managing risk of depression created by the organisation. Improved quality of data is needed to make that case as reliable data would aid objectivity and improve communication and understanding. Focused risk management strategies could then be devised to reduce the risk of occupationally induced ill health.

Government ultimately pays most of the cost of depressive illness, compounded if the person leaves employment to live on benefit payments. Further research into financial and medical risk management models in the workplace is urgently needed, as we currently understand little of how such models work at present. We need to develop a research base working across disciplines and working with employers and trade unions. This research should identify the most cost-effective, socially and medically appropriate interventions that keep people safely at work.

For their part, healthcare professionals need to work more closely with employers and occupational health practitioners on a case-by-case basis, and treat depression more urgently and effectively, with patients' future economic welfare paramount. If they become unemployed their mental state may deteriorate.[7] The depressed employee, at the centre of a complex web of roles, responsibilities and financial accountabilities, lies vulnerable. We must all work in a more co-ordinated way to prevent unnecessary unemployment. If we can achieve this then individuals can remain autonomous and productive, organisations can become even more effective, and the state should pay less in social and health costs.

References

1. Jones ME, Sutherland G. *Implementing Turnbull, A Boardroom Briefing*. London: Institute of Chartered Accountants, 1999.
2. *Good Health is Good Business: employers' guide* (Phase 3). MISC130, London: Health and Safety Executive, 1999.
3. *Goodwin v Patent Office* (1999) ICR 302.
4. *Walker v Northumberland County Council* (1995) 1 AER 737.
5. Kasl S, Amick B. Work Stress. In: McDonald, J C, ed. *Epidemiology of Work Related Disease*. London: BMJ Publishing Group, 1995.
6. http://www.infotech-wellness.com/index.html
7. Lewis G, Sloggett A. Suicide, deprivation and unemployment: record linkage study. *BMJ* 1998;317:1283–6.

Economic and Societal Consequences

Overview

The costs of clinical depression are easily identifiable but other costs are not so evident, such as the cost of family input. Twenty-five per cent of the severely depressed will attempt suicide, 15% will succeed. Whether or not the attempt succeeds there will be a cost to the family and to the community. In 1991, a United Kingdom National Health Service (NHS) study showed that the burden of dealing with neuroses was £900 million per year, or £16 for every man, woman and child; estimated at today's prices that would be in excess of £2 billion. The financial implications for the individual and the societal cost of lost human capital are rarely calculated. From the individual's point of view, the importance of diagnosing and properly treating depression in childhood and adolescence cannot be overemphasised. The tools for doing so are already available. In the workplace, temporary absenteeism causes a major loss of productivity potential. In the United Kingdom, the Confederation of British Industry has estimated that temporary absenteeism costs business over £10 billion each year of which depression accounts for a fair share.

Depression needs to be destigmatised. Anecdotally, it is easier to find employment for an ex-convict than for someone with a history of depression. These problems are covered in the first article.

The next two articles deal with the economic aspects of drug therapy. Over the past decade prescribing patterns have followed similar lines in that tricyclic antidepressants (TCAs), which were in vogue in the early 1990s, have given way to the newer selective serotonin-reuptake inhibitors (SSRIs). The first article from Canada, describes five distinct methodological techniques for assessing the economic outcomes associated with the use of antidepressant pharmacotherapy and considers the

119

strengths and weaknesses of each process. The second article reviews in more detail the prescribing patterns of antidepressants in several different countries and highlights the fact that patients are, for the most part, receiving suboptimal treatment for their depression, which is detrimental for the patient but also has massive economic implications for health services worldwide.

The economic consequences of depression

DANIEL CHISHOLM

Introduction: the epidemiological burden of depression

Depression is one of the most common psychiatric disorders and constitutes a significant public health burden as a result of its high prevalence, long duration, likelihood of recurrence, underdiagnosis and inadequate treatment.[1] An accumulating body of evidence has emerged, particularly since the mid-1990s onwards, that clearly demonstrates the massive, and previously underestimated, burden that depression imposes upon individuals, families and whole communities throughout the world.[2-4] This 'burden' of depression has been measured from a clinical or epidemiological perspective in terms of disability effects, levels of morbidity and mortality rates. There is substantial evidence to indicate that persons with depression suffer from a number of functional limitations, including poorer physical, psychosocial and role functioning and an increased number of disability days.[5-7] It has also been estimated that 15% of all patients with a major depressive disorder die by suicide.[8]

A notable attempt to capture both the mortality effects and the disabling consequences of disease was undertaken by the Global Burden of Disease study,[4] a key finding of which was that by combining the mortality and disability effects of disease into a single metric (the Disability Adjusted Life Year or DALY), the immense burden of global disease attributable to neuropsychiatric disorders became readily apparent. Depression is estimated to be the fourth largest contributor to the global burden of disease (3.7% of all causes), and by 2020 is projected to become the single largest in developing regions, owing to high prevalence rates (particularly among women), non-detection (90% in some regions) and severity (a disability weight of 0.6 out of 1 in untreated form).

Table 4 The burden of depression: a cost matrix.

	A. Care costs	B. Productivity costs	C. Other costs
1. Depressed individuals	Treatment and service fees/payments	Work disability Lost earnings	Anguish/suffering, treatment side effects, suicide
2. Family and friends	Informal care-giving	Time off work	Carer burden
3. Employers	Contributions to treatment and care	Reduced productivity	—
4. Society	Provision of mental health and general medical care (taxation/insurance)	Reduced productivity	Loss of lives, untreated depression (unmet need)

The economic burden of depression

The burden or consequences of depression can also be usefully gauged from an economic perspective. Depression imposes a range of costs on individuals, households, employers and on society as a whole (Table 4). A proportion of these costs are financially self-evident, including the varied contributions made by depressed individuals, employers and taxpayers/insurers towards the considerable costs of treatment and care (cells A1, A3, A4), and the productivity losses resulting from work disability, reduced attendance and impaired work performance (B1–B4). There are a series of further costs, however, which although not so readily quantifiable nevertheless represent very significant economic or opportunity costs. These include informal care inputs by family members and friends (A2), the suffering, treatment side effects and mortality among people with depression (C1) and the hidden societal cost of untreated depression (C4).

Table 5 The burden of depression: cost of illness studies.

Authors	Location, year	Direct costs	Indirect costs	Total costs	Ratio direct:indirect
• Kind and Sorensen (1993)[9]	UK, 1991	£417m	£2.97bn	£3.39bn	12:88
• Greenberg et al. (1993)[10]	USA, 1990	$12.4bn	$31.3bn	$43.7bn	28:72
• Rice and Miller (1995)[11]	USA, 1990	$19.8bn	$10.5bn	$30.4bn	65:35

The overall economic burden associated with depression and affective disorders has been estimated in a series of 'cost of illness' studies, which attempt to attach monetary values to these various societal costs (Table 5). Where a comprehensive cost estimate has been attempted, total estimated costs amount to £3.4 billion in the United Kingdom, and $30–40 billion in the United States (1990 price levels).[9-11] A common feature of these studies is that costs due to mortality and lost productivity constitute a very significant proportion of the total cost. This is in part due to the method used for calculating lost productivity, which assumes that all lost days of an adult's working life should be valued. In prevailing conditions of unemployment, this 'human capital' method represents an overestimation of true opportunity costs. An alternative basis for such computations is the 'friction-cost method', which only takes into account the productivity lost before a replacement worker is found. Applying this method to the costs of schizophrenia in Canada, the cost of lost productivity resulting from mortality was $1.53 million, as opposed to $105 million if the human-capital approach had been used.[12] In a less comprehensive but comparative cost of illness study in the United Kingdom, the NHS Executive demonstrated the *relative* magnitude of depression costs (Figure 2).[13] Costs to the NHS for neurotic disorders amounted to £887 million in 1992–93, exceeded only by psychotic disorders (£1159 million) and considerably greater than, for example, diabetes (£300 million) or hypertension (£439 million).

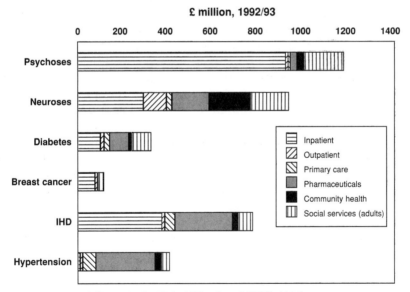

Figure 2 Burdens of disease in the United Kingdom (NHSE, 1996)

As with epidemiological projections such as the Global Burden of Disease study,[4] and despite methodological discrepancies, cost of illness studies clearly demonstrate the magnitude of the costs of depression. As such, they provide a useful context within which to investigate interventions or strategies that are capable of making an impact on this identified burden in terms of clinical and cost effectiveness.

Economic issues in the treatment of depression

Cost-effectiveness of pharmacological and psychotherapeutic interventions

Since the advent of tricyclic antidepressants (TCAs), the treatment of depression has been dominated by pharmacotherapy. This seems set to continue in the light of recent technological developments, notably the introduction of a new class of antidepressant drugs, selective serotonin-reuptake inhibitors (SSRIs), which are widely accepted to have at least equivalent efficacy as TCAs but a lower risk of toxicity and adverse side-effects, arguably leading to greater compliance and consequent reductions in use of health and other services. Against this, the newer SSRIs carry considerably higher acquisition costs. There is consequently an important cost-effectiveness question to be considered: are the higher acquisition costs of SSRIs worth paying for in terms of the reduced toxicity, adverse side effects and need for service inputs that they bring to patients? Until further data are generated from prospective cost-effectiveness studies undertaken in the context of primary care settings, it is only currently possible to conclude that there is no definitive evidence that demonstrates clear dominance (both in terms of costs and outcomes) for either treatment strategy.[14] (For a review of evidence, see the article by David Sclar, p.143).

Whilst the key cost-effectiveness debate has centred around antidepressant drugs, there have been a small number of studies that have explored the relative cost-effectiveness of psychotherapeutic interventions in the treatment of depression. One recent controlled trial concluded that economic costs and quality of life outcomes for primary care patients receiving interpersonal therapy were superior to usual care (though slightly inferior to those assigned to receive pharmacotherapy), and assuming a unit cost per session of 80% or less of the Medicare reimbursement rate, represented a cost-effective intervention (against the benchmark threshold of $20 000 per Quality Adjusted Life Year).[15] There is a need for further prospective studies with sufficient sample sizes and cost coverage to definitively address the cost-effectiveness of these alternative interventions.

Under-recognition of depression

A critical issue in the management of depression is non-detection. In a recent six-country survey in Europe, nearly 60% of those with major depression received no treatment.[16] The majority of these people did not even seek treatment for their symptoms, and only a quarter received an antidepressant. High rates of non-detection were also reported in the WHO study of psychological problems in general healthcare.[2] Failure to detect cases is largely attributable to misdiagnosis due to concurrence of other symptoms or somatic disorders, the physical expression of depressive symptoms (somatisation), or factors relating to the consultation process (such as clinical expertise or patient trust). This indicates that there has been a massive underestimation of the economic impact of depression internationally.

The costs of *not* treating depression in the United States were considered by Rupp,[17] who performed a 'what-if?' scenario to analyse the changes in costs of depression that would result from an increase of adequate treatment to 70% of all depression cases, and concluded that the direct costs of care and treatment in the United States would increase by $4.2 billion, but mortality and morbidity costs would each decrease by over $4.2 billion, giving an overall 'saving' of $4.1bn to society. In a similar vein, the Global Burden of Disease study[4] estimated that 8.4% (out of 83 million) episodes of depression in the developing world receive treatment compared to 35% in developed regions. Increasing the rate of treatment to that currently achieved in more developed regions would therefore reduce the burden of illness due to depression in the developing world by 13%, saving 5.7 million DALYs per year (Michael Phillips, personal communication).

Suboptimal prescribing and non-compliance

Even when a patient has been correctly diagnosed, adequacy of treatment is not assured. Recommended dosages of antidepressants and treatment guidelines for depression are widely available but may not be heeded owing to the side-effect profiles of these medications or insufficient monitoring by practitioners of appropriate therapeutic levels and/or duration. Subtherapeutic prescribing of antidepressants appears to be highly prevalent, particularly for the older TCAs.[16, 18] This not only has educational implications for primary care doctors, but is also likely to be associated with poorer outcomes, leading in turn to greater use of health and social care services. Patients may also interrupt their treatment, which unless the depression is naturally resolving, is likely to increase relapse and lead to higher medical resource consumption in the long term. One study concluded that a treatment failure was associated with an increase of over US$1000 over a one-year period in medical costs.[19]

Locus and quality of care

Using data from the Medical Outcomes Study, Sturm and Wells demonstrated that, although treatment for depression in the mental health specialist sector is more expensive than treatment in the general medical sector, it also leads to greater improvements in functional outcomes and represents the more cost-effective strategy (Figure 3).[5] Similarly, Zhang *et al.*[20] show that while the expected costs of treatment for the average patient receiving depression treatment in the mental health sector were $1224 higher than that in the general medical sector, lost earnings were $2101 lower (a net saving of $887 per patient per year). Measurement of total healthcare costs is important because of the possibility that, in the long run, mental healthcare may reduce general medical expenditures. A review of this 'cost-offset' effect concluded that although a number of cross-sectional and quasi-experimental studies support an association between depression and medical utilisation, there are no experimental studies that clearly establish that such a cost-offset can be realised.[21]

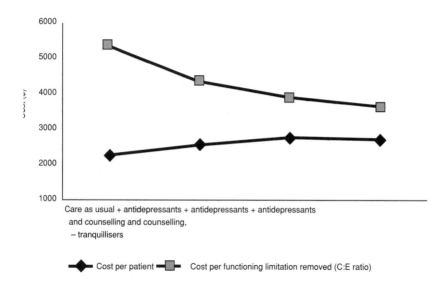

Figure 3 Improving the quality and cost-effectiveness of treatment for depression (Sturm and Wells, 1995)

Conclusion: the need for evidence-based investment

The increasing recognition of mental health as a significant international public health issue has led to additional demands for resources that are already stretched:[3]

Economic constraints, particularly those resulting from mandated efforts to restructure economies, have placed extreme limits on governments' abilities to develop new services or extend successful programmes. In the context of scarcity, mental health services are seldom given high priority

126

by national governments or by international aid programmes. The importance of addressing the wide-ranging problems [associated with] mental and behavioural problems ... should be recognised as crucial for both human and economic development.

There is therefore a requirement to demonstrate that investment is needed and worthwhile, which translates into generating evidence on affordable and cost-effective mental healthcare and prevention strategies. Alongside efforts to raise political will and public awareness, such an evidence base is an important step in impressing on governments that additional mental health resources (most notably in training, effective psychotropic drugs and basic infrastructures), can generate significant health gain and other benefits. Unfortunately, however, there is currently a dearth of cost and outcome data upon which to base these decisions in most regions of the world, which poses an awkward predicament, namely that despite the abundance of epidemiological and clinical evidence pointing to the need for investment, there is a paucity of economic evidence to guide or support these investment decisions.

Table 6 Cost-effectiveness questions in the management of depression.

Level of economic development	Prevailing features of mental health system	Cost-effectiveness research priorities in the management of depression
Developed regions (e.g. North America, Western Europe)	Relatively well-resourced; market-based reforms; community-based services; new psychotropic drugs	Comparison between older and newer anti-depressants and psychotherapeutic interventions Evaluation of the impact of managed or shared care reforms on the cost and quality of care
Developing regions (e.g. East and West Africa, South Asia)	Very poorly resourced; low policy priority; very limited access to services	Integration of mental health into primary healthcare training and practice Evaluation of the impact of widening the availability of low-cost antidepressants Mobilisation of local resources (e.g. indigenous healers) Demonstration of the need for investment into mental healthcare

The precise information requirements for policy development obviously need to reflect local or regional realities and levels of economic development; for example, assessing the relative cost-effectiveness of older versus newer antidepressants is unlikely to represent a high priority concern in countries where the availability of *any* antidepressants is at issue. Nevertheless, a number of broad areas where economic evidence appears to be particularly warranted in industrialised and low-income countries can be identified (Table 6). Such economic studies ideally need to incorporate a comparative perspective (for example, by including single index measures of outcome such as Quality Adjusted or Disability Adjusted Life Years), so that policymakers can make informed resource allocation decisions across alternative programmes of healthcare investment.

Addressing this research agenda represents a substantial challenge, not least because there are currently so many gaps and because findings generated in one particular setting or country cannot be readily generalised to others, owing to the heterogeneity of healthcare systems. However, the large number of completed studies with positive or encouraging findings (mainly in the United States), together with the broad methodological consensus that has been reached in the application of economic evaluation to healthcare, holds out the prospect of a new generation of studies that are capable of demonstrating that interventions for depression in diverse cultural settings are affordable, effective and can be expected to lead not only to improvements in health but also to the greater productivity of individuals, households and communities alike.

References

1. Bland RC. Epidemiology of affective disorders: a review. *Can J Psychiatry* 1997;**42**:367–77.
2. Üstün TB, Sartorius N, eds. *Mental Illness in General Health*. Chichester: John Wiley, 1995.
3. Desjarlais R, Eisenberg L, Good B, Kleinman A. *World Mental Health: problems and priorities in low-income countries*. New York: Oxford University Press, 1995.
4. Murray CJL, Lopez AD, eds. *The Global Burden of Disease*. Cambridge, MA: Harvard University Press, 1995.
5. Sturm R, Wells KB. How can care for depression become more cost-effective? *JAMA* 1995;**273**:51–8.
6. Von Korff M, Ormel J, Katon W, Lin EH. Disability and depression among high utilizers of healthcare: a longitudinal analysis. *Arch Gen Psychiatry* 1992;**49**: 91–100.
7. Broadhead WE, Blazer DG, George LK, Tse CK. Depression, disability days and days lost from work in a prospective epidemiologic survey. *JAMA* 1990;**264**:2524–28.
8. Guze SB, Robins E. Suicide and primary affective disorders. *Br J Psychiatry*, 1970;**117**:437–8.
9. Kind P, Sorensen J. The costs of depression. *Int Clin Psychopharmacol* 1993;**7**:191–5.
10. Greenberg PE, Stiglin LE, Finkelstein SN, Berndt ER. The economic burden of depression in 1990. *J Clin Psychiatry* 1993;**54**:405–18.
11. Rice DP, Miller LS. The economic burden of affective disorders. *Br J Psychiatry* (Suppl) 1995;**166**:34–42.
12. Goeree R, O'Brien B, Goering P *et al.* The economic burden of schizophrenia in Canada. *Can J Psychiatry* 1999;**44**:464–72.
13. Department of Health. NHS Executive. *Burdens of Disease*. Leeds: Department of Health, 1996.
14. Woods SW, Baker CB. Cost-effectiveness of newer antidepressants. *Curr Opin Psychiatry* 1997;**10**:95–101.
15. Lave JR, Frank RG, Shulberg HC, Kamlet MS. Cost-effectiveness of treatments for major depression in primary care practice. *Arch Gen Psychiatry* 1998;**55**:645–51.

16. Lepine JP, Gastpar M, Mendlewicz J, Tylee A. Depression in the community: the first pan-European study DEPRES (Depression Research in European Society). *Int Clin Psychopharmacol* 1997;**12**:19–29.
17. Rupp A. The economic consequences of not treating depression. *Br J Psychiatry Suppl* 1995;**166**:29–33.
18. Donoghue JM, Tylee A. The treatment of depression: prescribing patterns of antidepressants in primary care in the United Kingdom. *Br J Psychiatry* 1996;**168**:164–8.
19. McCombs JS, Nichols MB. The cost of treatment failure. In: Jonsson B, Rosenbaum J, eds. *Health Economics of Depression*. Chichester: John Wiley, 1993.
20. Zhang M, Rost KM, Fortney JC. Earnings changes for depressed individuals treated by mental health specialists. *Am J Psychiatry* 1999;**156**:108–14.
21. Simon GE, Katzelnick DJ. Depression, use of medical services and cost-offset effects. *J Psychsom Res* 1997;**42**:333–44.

Reducing the costs of depression: opportunities in the millennium

ERNST R BERNDT

The burden of depression is a staggering one. Among the components contributing to this burden, medical treatment costs are substantial, but non-medical costs are much larger. Within the medical cost component, research from US retrospective medical claims data indicates that about 25% of the annual direct medical costs of a typical patient being treated for depression are depression-related costs, while the remaining 75% are from other, often somatic, co-morbidities[1]. However, a number of studies have shown that the non-medical or indirect costs of depression are several times larger than the direct medical costs. These indirect costs include impaired ability to function, reduced productivity at work, increased absenteeism, and, to a much smaller extent, mortality from suicide.[2–9] While not treating depression may save on medical costs (depending on whether depression treatment costs would be offset by reduced non-depression-related medical costs), the indirect costs persist and constitute an enormous burden even when depression is not treated.[10–11] That depression is undertreated and frequently misdiagnosed is now a well-documented phenomenon.[12–16]

One way of quantifying the burden of these largely non-medical costs is through a measure of Disability Adjusted Life Years (DALYs) — the number of years lost to morbidity and mortality. A recent study conducted by the World Health Organization and the World Bank finds that among all people between ages 15–44 years in the world in 1990, unipolar major depression alone accounted for more than 10% of all DALYs, making it the leading cause of disease burden (Table 7)[17].

While the burden of depression is a staggering one, its indirect cost component can be reduced significantly with antidepressant treatment.

Evidence now documents a clear relationship between clinical and functional outcomes: as the clinical symptoms of depression improve following treatment, so does the ability to function at work and at home[18]. Moreover, the work outcome response for clinical responders is substantial, rapid and sustainable.

Table 7 Ten leading causes of Disability Adjusted Life Years (DALYs) Ages 15–44 years 1990 (after Murray and Lopez, 1996).[17]

		DALYs (in thousands)		
Rank	Disease or injury	Males	Females	Total
1	Unipolar major depression	15321	27651	42972
2	Tuberculosis	10937	8736	19673
3	Road traffic accidents	15554	4072	19626
4	Alcohol use	13096	1752	14848
5	Self-inflicted injuries	7550	7095	14645
6	Bipolar disorder	6736	6453	13189
7	War	7899	5235	13134
8	Violence	11040	1915	12955
9	Schizophrenia	6646	5896	12542
10	Iron deficiency anaemia	5003	7508	12511

Evidence linking symptomatic and functional improvements

Let me describe some of this economic evidence from a recently completed randomised double-blind clinical trial, whose principal clinical findings are discussed elsewhere[19-22]. The trial involved 635 chronically depressed patients (DSM-III-R-defined chronic major or double depression) at baseline, and consisted of a 12-week acute phase with a 12-week crossover phase for acute-phase non-responders, a 16-week continuation phase for those responding at week 12, and a 76-week maintenance phase. Based on symptomatic metrics such as the Hamilton Depression Rating Scale and the Clinical Global Impression of Improvement, patients receiving the antidepressant sertraline were categorised either as full responders, partial responders or non-responders. A number of other instruments were employed to measure psychosocial functioning, and to compare scores of clinical trial subjects with those from 'normal populations', based on community studies.

One instrument used to assess ability to function was the well-known Medical Outcomes Study Health Status Questionnaire, Short Form 36-item (SF-36) survey[23]. In Figure 4, scores of Social Functioning subscale of the SF-36 are on the vertical axis (Best = 100, population norm = 82.7), while various observation points during the two-year trial are on the horizontal axis. The vertical bars display average SF-36 scores separately for full, partial and non-responders. Three points are worth noting from Figure 4[24]. First, substantial improvement in social functioning occurs for all three groups, but is largest for the full responders (based on clinical symptoms). By acute week 12, social functioning scores are highest for the full responders (slightly higher than population norms), at 80.1, are about the same as population norms for the partial responders, and are even significantly improved for those judged to be clinical non-responders (from 49.8 at baseline to 75.3 at week 12). Second, the improvement in social functioning is rapid. Already by week 4, average scores are significantly different from baseline ($p \leq$ 0.001 for each of the three groups), and improvements continue to week 12. Third, the improvements in social functioning are sustained. From acute week 12 to maintenance week 76, there is no significant change in the mean social functioning test scores, for both partial and full responders. To summarise, the functional improvement for clinical responders is substantial, rapid and sustained, and this improvement is even significant for clinical non-responders.

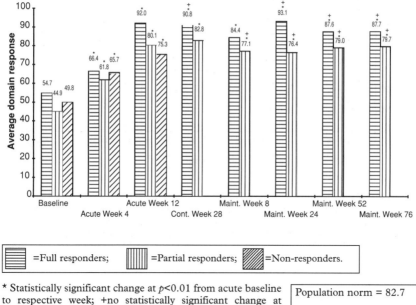

=Full responders;   =Partial responders;   =Non-responders.

* Statistically significant change at $p<0.01$ from acute baseline to respective week; +no statistically significant change at $p>0.01$ from acute week 12 to respective week. Sample size is indicated by the number at the bottom of each respective bar. Cont. = continuation; Maint. = maintenance.

Population norm = 82.7

S.D. = 22.5

Figure 4 SF-36: Social Functioning (Best=100).

Another outcome measure reflecting the reduced societal burden when depressives receive treatment involves their ability and energy to go to work. In this same clinical trial lasting two years, responders to sertraline at continuation week 28 were randomised to placebo or sertraline treatment. As seen in Figure 5, before randomisation but after about half a year of sertraline treatment, the average number of hours worked in the past two weeks (for those working that respective week, as reported in Question #5h of the Social Adjustment Scale – Self Report instrument[25]) increased by about 13% from 67.4 at baseline to 76.3 at continuation week 28. Following randomisation at continuation week 28, average hours worked by those subjects randomised to sertraline remained essentially unchanged at 78.4 at maintenance week 24; for those randomised to placebo, however, average hours worked fell significantly to 62.8 at maintenance week 24, and even further to 53.0 and 50.5 at maintenance weeks 52 and 76, respectively.

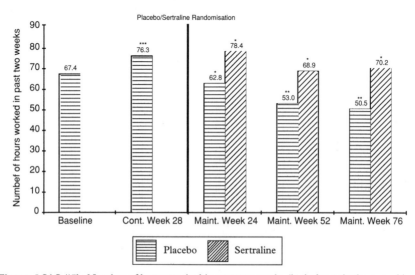

Figure 5 SAS #5h: Number of hours worked in past two weeks (includes only those working that respective week). *** Statistically significant change at $p<0.01$ from baseline to continuation (Cont.) week 28; **, * statistically significant change at $p<0.01$ and 0.05 respectively from continuation week 28 to respective maintenance (Maint.) week; +no statistically significant change at $p>0.01$ from continuation week 28 to respective maintenance week. Sample size is indicated by the number at the bottom of each respective bar.

In summary, responders to antidepressant treatment manifest not only symptomatic improvement, but also functional improvement. Since a very substantial portion of the burden of depression involves functional impairment, treatment of chronic depressives with antidepressants can reduce this societal burden considerably.

Opportunities for reducing the burden of depression

Although treatment with antidepressants is efficacious, there is much room for improvement. In randomised controlled trials, first-line antidepressant pharmacotherapy typically achieves 50–60% full remission rates, and after multiple lines of antidepressant pharmacotherapy, remission rates of 65–80% are often attained.[15,20,26–27] This implies that 20–35% of patients do not respond to antidepressant pharmacotherapy. In the naturalistic setting, it is likely that remission rates are even lower than this, due to patient non-compliance and attrition. I will return to this point later.

Where are the largest opportunities for reducing the societal costs of depression? One way to think about this is to ask, who receives antidepressant drug therapy today? Based on National Disease and Therapeutic Index market data from IMS America, it appears that about 75% of those receiving antidepressant drug therapy are between the ages of 20 and 59, 19% are age 60 or older, and only 6% are under age 20. The vast majority of those being prescribed antidepressants, therefore, are in the working ages between 20 and 59. I now focus on both the youngest and the oldest segments, and outline opportunities for reducing the societal costs of depression among these less treated age groups.

Early onset major depressive disorder and lost human capital

Epidemiological research has shown that the prevalence of major depressive disorder to age 24 is 21% for females and 11% for males, and to age 21 is 15% vs 8%[28]. A striking finding from this literature is that the median age of onset of major depressive disorder is about 21 — half of mature adults who at some time were depressed had their initial onset before age 21. While the prevalence of early onset depression is surprisingly high, diagnosing depression reliably in young patients presents challenges, particularly since mood changes are normal among adolescents. Clearly there is potential both for undertreatment and overtreatment, and reliable diagnosis and early intervention are critical.

Additional insight on the prevalence and consequences of early onset depression emerged from the same clinical trial I discussed earlier. This clinical evidence is consistent with the epidemiological literature. Moreover, it illustrates that the societal costs of early onset depression are very, very substantial. Specifically, the trial involved 635 subjects, all diagnosed with chronic depression. We partitioned the subjects to those over and those under age 30 at baseline, and found that 43% of the older subjects had early onset (before age 22) major depressive disorder, roughly what one would expect based on epidemiological evidence. An interesting and significant clinical finding was that there was no difference in antidepressant efficacy among early versus late onset depressives.[29]

However, one important difference between the early and late onset older depressives was their educational attainment. Since most individuals complete their post-secondary schooling by age 30, by focusing on those trial subjects over age 30 at baseline, we were able to examine differential

135

educational attainment histories of early versus late onset depressives. For males, we found no significant differences in educational attainment between the early and late onset depressives. We also found no differences in the probability of going to college among early and late onset depressives, male or female. However, given college attendance, early onset females were only 57% as likely as late onset females to complete college ($p \leq 0.05$). Further, among those who obtained a college degree, early onset females were only 50% as likely as late onset females to obtain a postgraduate degree ($p \leq 0.10$). For young females, therefore, one important consequence of early onset depression is the impaired ability to accumulate human capital in the form of additional schooling. In the parlance of economics, for young females the 'lost human capital' of early onset major depressive disorder is substantial, and can be mitigated.

One way of quantifying this societal cost of lost human capital is to ask: suppose we randomly chose two 21-year-old women in 1995, one with early onset depression, and the other either a late onset or never depressive. Because early onset depression impairs educational attainment, which in turn affects future earnings prospects in the workplace, what would be the difference in expected annual earnings of these two 21-year-old females as they age? The results of such a calculation, based on integrated US Census schooling and earnings data, and data from the clinical trial, are presented in Figure 6.[29] A randomly chosen 21-year-old female with early onset major depressive disorder in 1995 can expect at age 35 to earn about 12% less ($19795 vs. $22461) than a randomly chosen 21-year-old female with late

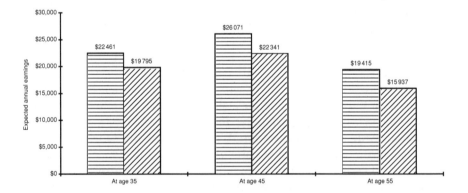

Figure 6 Effect of age of onset on expected mean annual earnings through lost human capital accumulation (results of logistic labour force participation and least squares earnings regressions). ▤ = Females with depression onset after age 21 or never; ▨ = early onset females. The prevalence of early onset major depression for females is assumed to be 15%. (Source Berndt *et al.*[29].)

or never onset depression. This difference grows to about 14% at age 45 ($26 071 vs. $22 341), and to 18% at age 55 ($15 937 vs $19 415). These earnings differentials reflect the relatively impaired ability of early versus late onset depressives to accumulate human capital in the form of additional years of schooling. An important implication is that there is a very substantial opportunity to reduce the societal costs of depression by diagnosing and appropriately treating adolescents and young adults, particularly young females.

Depression among the elderly: opportunities and challenges

Additional opportunities to reduce the burden of depression involve treatment of the elderly. This opportunity emerges in part because people are living longer today, with many having either survived or avoided other somatic illnesses. Moreover, while still a powerful force to reckon with, the stigma of major depressive disorder is likely to be reduced gradually as the 'baby-boom' cohort ages. But diagnosing depression in the elderly is challenging, particularly since geriatric co-morbidities are more prevalent than in the young, and since some of the symptoms of depression commonly observed in younger adults (e.g. sleep disturbances), when observed in the elderly may instead be associated with conditions and disorders other than depression. Evaluating the benefits of treatment in the elderly presents additional challenges, such as how one weights Quality Adjusted Life Years in the elderly, especially among retirees and those institutionalised.[30-32]

Hence, the opportunities for reducing the costs of depression among the elderly via more effective diagnosis and treatment are substantial, but so too are the challenges.

Themes and counterthemes in the millennium: reducing the costs of depression

With this as background, I now turn to a discussion of various themes and counterthemes concerning opportunities for reducing the burden of depression in the new millennium. Here I discuss four sets of issues.

First, the undertreatment of depression in the young and in the elderly offers enormous opportunity to reduce the societal costs of this disorder. But reliably diagnosing and appropriately treating depression in adolescents, and perhaps even more so in geriatric patients, presents enormous challenges. Will effective and reliable diagnoses in these patient age segments require psychiatric specialists, or will primary care physicians be trained better to diagnose and treat the young and the elderly? To the extent specialty training will be required, the increased use of non-specialist gatekeepers in managed medical care may constrain considerably the potential growth in treatment for depression, and thereby impair our ability to reduce the societal costs of this disorder.

Second, there is mounting recent clinical trial evidence that combining targeted forms of psychotherapy along with antidepressant pharmacotherapy achieves higher remission rates than does either monotherapy for the treatment of depression or Dysthymia.[33-35] What is not clear, however, is whether the targeted psychotherapy used in combination treatments requires specialised psychiatric training, training and tools not in the typical toolkit of general practitioners, family practitioners, and internists. Can the psychotherapy be implemented effectively by non-specialists? Will less-structured group therapy in combination with pharmacotherapy be more successful than either monotherapy? I submit that the appropriate training for and use of combination therapies offers major challenges both to academic medicine and to providers – managed care and others.

Third, the success of the selective serotonin-reuptake inhibitors (SSRIs) in replacing tricyclic antidepressants (TCAs) as first-line therapies has been remarkable in the United States, albeit not as dramatic yet in Europe. This success is due in large part to the 'user friendliness' of the SSRIs – they are safe and patients can tolerate them better than the TCAs. But as I noted earlier, at least 20–35% of depressives still do not respond to multiple lines of antidepressant drug therapy. What will it take to obtain more satisfactory and effective antidepressant drug treatment? The physicians and psychiatrists with whom I interact typically place three items on their antidepressant drug 'most wanted' list: (i) greater, or more selective, targeted efficacy; (ii) more rapid onset of treatment response; and (iii) reduced side effects, particularly those involving sexual dysfunction.

Fourth, given current knowledge, there is no reason to expect that one single new drug, or even a single new drug class involving distinct mechanisms of action, will meet these various needs – the depressive illnesses are complex and multifaceted. What is needed, therefore, to make a major dent in reducing the burden of depression, is the discovery and development of a substantial number of new antidepressant drugs. For that to occur, however, incentives need to be in place for the research and development that is necessary to discover and develop new antidepressants.

Demand management and increases in mental health expenditures

There are many who believe, however, that the discovery and development of new antidepressants will only increase even further the ever-growing expenditures for the treatment of depression. Now it may well be that because of the complexity of their illness, those now unresponsive to antidepressant pharmacotherapy may require new and more costly treatments. But it is also critically important to examine more generally the causes and sources of growing mental health expenditures.

In the United States and in many other countries in recent years, expenditures on mental healthcare have been increasing. But why? Is the increase in expenditures due to the increasing cost per episode of treatment for the mental illness? Or is it due to the increasing number of episodes of mental illness that are being treated? Or is it some combination of these two? Note that expenditures is the multiplicative product of cost per illness episode times the number of illness episodes treated.

Using a large retrospective United States medical claims' database covering more than 600 000 lives, together with some colleagues at the Harvard Medical School I have recently been examining time trends in the cost of treating an episode of major depressive disorder with treatment that is consistent with the AHCPR guidelines.[27] The results suggest that over the 1991–96 period, the cost of guideline-consistent treatment for an episode of major depressive disorder has been falling at about 3% per year, in large part because increased use of antidepressant drugs has been accompanied by less intensive use of psychotherapy.[36–38] With treatment cost per episode falling by around 3% per year and with total expenditures for the treatment of episodes increasing over the same period, the clear implication is that the number of depressive disorders being treated has been increasing substantially. This is welcome news, for it means that the reason medical mental health spending for depression is increasing is because more people are being treated, thereby reducing the overall societal cost of this illness.

Some final thoughts

Where then shall we look to reduce the societal burden of major depressive disorder? I believe the evidence shows that we are focusing too much on the medical costs of treating depression, and are overlooking the enormous reduction in the non-medical costs of this illness that accompany treatment with antidepressants – reductions in work impairment and in impaired ability to function. We can point our fingers and focus our eyes on rising treatment expenditures, but that is I believe the wrong place to look if we really want to reduce the overall cost of this illness. To reduce the societal costs of treated and currently untreated depression, it may well be necessary to increase medical expenditures further, even as the average cost of treating an episode of depression has been declining in the United States.

Where shall we look to reduce the societal costs of depression in the millennium? The cost of medications is large, but these costs must be reckoned in relation to the benefits of treatment, particularly the much larger reductions in the non-medical burdens from depression that accompany treatment. Today we have a much larger and varied set of antidepressant pharmacotherapies to treat depression effectively, and in recent years we have gained new knowledge of more effective blends of psychotherapy and pharmacotherapy. But new medications are needed, for a substantial portion of depressives do not respond to currently available treatments – and the non-medical costs of these depressives is not only large, but can some day be reduced as well.

The record of drug discovery and innovation in the last few decades is powerful evidence showing that research and development responds to perceived opportunities that in turn foster innovation. To reduce the overall societal burden of depression, public and private payers need to signal credibly a willingness to pay for the next generation of antidepressant treatments.

References

1. Russell JM, Berndt ER, Miceli RM *et al*. Course and cost of treatment for depression with fluoxetine, paroxetine and sertraline. *Am J Manag Care* 1999;5:597–606.
2. Greenberg PE, Stiglin LE, Finkelstein SN, Berndt ER. The economic burden of depression in 1990. *J Clin Psychiatry* 1993;54:405–18.
3. Greenberg PE, Stiglin LE, Finkelstein SN, Berndt ER. Depression: a neglected major illness. *J Clin Psychiatry* 1993;54:419–24.
4. Greenberg PE, Kessler RC, Nells TL *et al*. Depression in the workplace: an economic perspective. In: Feighner JP, Boyers WF, eds. *Selective Serotonin Reuptake Inhibitors: advances in basic research and clinical practice*, pp.327–63. Chichester: John Wiley, 1996.
5. Kind P, Sorenson J. The costs of depression. *Int Clin Psychopharmacol* 1993;7:191-5.
6. Jonsson B, Bebbington PE. What price depression? The cost of depression and the cost-effectiveness of pharmacological treatment. *Br J Psychiatry* 1994;164:665–73.
7. Conti DJ, Burton WN. The economic impact of depression in a workplace. *J Occup Med* 1994;36:983–8.
8. Wells KB, Stewart A, Hays RD *et al*. The functioning and well-being of depressed patients. Results from the medical outcomes study. *JAMA* 1989;262:914–9.
9. Schonfeld WH, Verboncoeur CJ, Fifer SK *et al*. The functioning and well-being of patients with unrecognized anxiety disorders and major depressive disorder. *J Affect Disord* 1997;43:105–19.
10. Simon GE, Katzelnick DJ. Depression, use of medical services and cost-offset effects. *J Psychosom Res* 1997;42:333–44.
11. Von Korff M, Katon W, Bush T *et al*. Treatment costs, cost offset and cost-effectiveness of collaborative management of depression. *Psychosom Med* 1998;60:143–9.
12. Keller MB, Lavori PW. The adequacy of treating depression. *J Nerv Ment Dis* 1988;176:471–4.
13. Katon W, Von Korff M, Lin EB *et al*. Adequacy and duration of antidepressant treatment in primary care. *Med Care* 1992;30:67–76.
14. Simon GE, Lin EB, Katon W *et al*. Outcomes of 'inadequate' antidepressant treatment. *J Gen Intern Med* 1995;10:663–70.
15. Regier DA, Hirschfeld RMA, Goodwin FK *et al*. The NIMH depression awareness, recognition, and treatment program: structure, aims, and scientific basis. *Am J Psychiatry* 1988;145:1351–57.
16. Lepine JP, Gastpar M, Mendlewicz J, Tylee A. Depression in the community: the first pan-European study. *Int Clin Psychopharmacol* 1997;12:19–29.
17. Murray CJ, Lopez AD, eds. *The Global Burden of Disease*. Cambridge, MA: Harvard University Press, 1996.
18. Berndt ER, Finkelstein SN, Greenberg PE *et al*. Workplace performance effects from chronic depression and its treatment. *J Health Econ* 1998;17:511–35.
19. Rush AJ, Koran LM, Keller MB *et al*. The treatment of chronic depression. Part 1. Study design and rationale for evaluating the comparative efficacy of sertraline and imipramine as acute, crossover, continuation, and maintenance phase therapies. *J Clin Psychiatry*

1998;**59**:589–97.

20. Keller MB, Gelenberg AJ, Hirschfeld RMA *et al.* The treatment of chronic depression, part 2. A double-blind, randomized trial of sertraline and imipramine. *J Clin Psychiatry* 1998;**59**:598–607.

21. Miller IW, Keitner GI, Schatzberg AF *et al.* The treatment of chronic depression. Part 3. Psychosocial functioning before and after treatment with sertraline or imipramine. *J Clin Psychiatry* 1998;**59**:608–19.

22. Kornstein SG, Schatzberg AF, Thase ME *et al.* Gender differences in chronic major and double depression. *J Affect Disord* 1998 (in press).

23. Ware JE Jr, Sherbourne CD. The MOS 36-item short-form health survey (SF-36). I. Conceptual framework and item selection. *Med Care* 1992;**30**:473–83.

24. Finkelstein SN, Berndt ER, Gelenberg AJ *et al.* 'Work-related outcomes during two years of sertraline therapy for chronic depression.' Manuscript, data on file. Cambridge, MA: Massachusetts Institute of Technology, Program on the Pharmaceutical Industry, 1999.

25. Weissman MM, Bothwell S. Assessment of social adjustment by patient self-report. *Arch Gen Psychiatry* 1976;**33**:1111–15.

26. American Psychiatric Association. Practice guideline for major depressive disorder in adults. *Am J Psychiatry* 1993;**150**:1a–26a.

27. Agency for Health Care Policy Research. *Depression in Primary Care, Vol. 2. Treatment of Major Depression, Clinical practice guideline; No. 5.* Rockville, MD: AHCPR, 1993.

28. Kessler RC, McGonagle KA, Swartz M *et al.* Sex and depression in the national comorbidity survey. I. lifetime prevalence, chronicity and recurrence. *J Affect Disord* 1993;**29**:85–96.

29. Berndt ER, Koran LM, Finkelstein SN *et al.* Lost human capital from early-onset chronic depression. *Am J Psychiatry* 2000;**157**:940–7.

30. Whalley D, McKenna SP. Measuring quality of life in patients with depression or anxiety. *Pharmacoeconomics* 1995;**8**:305–15.

31. Mesters P, Cosyns P, Dejaiffe G, *et al.* Assessment of quality of life in the treatment of major depressive disorder with fluoxetine, 20 mg, in ambulatory patients aged over 60 years. *Int Clin Psychopharmacol* 1993;**8**:337–40.

32. Lave JR, Frank RG, Schulberg HC, Kamlet MS. Cost-effectiveness of treatments for major depression in primary care practice. *Arch Gen Psychiatry* 1998;**55**:645–51.

33. Keller MB, McCullough JP, Klein DN *et al.* Nefazodone HCl, CBASP and combination therapy for the acute treatment of chronic depression. In: *Proceedings of the One Hundred and Fifty Second Annual Meeting of the American Psychiatric Association.* Washington, DC: American Psychiatric Association, 1999.

34. Keller MB, McCullough JP, Klein DN *et al.* The acute treatment of chronic major depression: a comparison of nefazodone, cognitive behavioral analysis system of psychotherapy, and their combination. *N Engl J Med* 2000;**342**:1462–70.

35. Ravindran AV, Anisman H, Merali Z *et al.* Treatment of primary dysthymia with group cognitive therapy and pharmacotherapy: clinical symptoms and functional impairments. *Am J Psychiatry* 1999;**156**:1608–17.

36. Frank RG, Busch SH, Berndt ER. Measuring prices and quantities of treatment for depression. *Am Econ Rev* 1998;**88**:106–11.

37. Frank RG, Berndt ER, Busch SH. Price indexes for the treatment of depression. In: Triplett JE, ed. *Measuring the Prices of Medical Treatments.* pp.72–117. Washington, DC: Brookings Institution 1999.

38. Berndt ER, Bir A, Busch SH *et al.* 'Productive inefficiency, price indexes and expected outcomes for treatment of depression.' Manuscript, data on file. Cambridge MA: Massachusetts Institute of Technology, Program on the Pharmaceutical Industry, 2000.

Economics of antidepressant pharmacotherapy: why SSRIs represent value for money

DAVID ALEXANDER SCLAR

Epidemiological studies hold that depressive disorders are among the most common forms of mental illness. Moreover, evidence suggests that there has been a significant increase in the prevalence of depression since the Second World War.[1] The National Comorbidity Survey has established the 30-day prevalence of major depression in the general population of the United States at approximately 5%, with a lifetime prevalence rate of approximately 17%[2]. An estimated $44 billion are expended annually in the United States for the treatment, morbidity, and mortality associated with depression.[3] By the year 2020 the global burden of depression is projected to rank second only to that of ischaemic heart disease.[4]

In the United States the number of office-based physician-patient encounters documenting a diagnosis of depression increased 23.2% between 1990 and 1995.[5] During this timeframe, the prescribing of tricyclic antidepressants (TCAs) declined from 42.1% in 1990, to 24.9% in 1995. In contrast, the use of a selective serotonin-reuptake inhibitor (SSRI) for the treatment of depression increased from 37.1% of encounters in 1990, to 64.6% in 1995. The rate of office-based encounters documenting the use of antidepressant pharmacotherapy for any purpose increased from 6.7 per 100 US population in 1990, to 10.9 in 1995, a 62.7% increase; documentation of a diagnosis of depression increased from 6.1 per 100 US population in 1990, to 7.1 in 1995, a 16.4% increase; and the recording of a diagnosis of depression in concert with the prescribing or continuation of antidepressant pharmacotherapy increased from 3.2 per 100 US population in 1990, to 4.8 in 1995, a 50% increase.

When correctly diagnosed and aggressively managed, depression is a highly treatable disease.[1] However, major depression remains an underdiagnosed and undertreated condition, with only one in three persons with depression pursuing treatment.[1,2] The persistent social stigma associated with depressive illness remains a major reason for its undertreatment.[2] Additionally, concomitant disease states, especially in the elderly, often obscure the diagnosis of depression, thereby leaving large numbers of patients untreated.[1,2]

Pharmacotherapy represents a first-line option in the management of major depressive illness. Recent pharmacotherapeutic advances in the treatment of patients with depression have included the development of the SSRIs, thereby providing an alternative to TCAs.[3] The SSRIs have achieved a rapid acceptance by prescribers worldwide due to an enhanced safety profile to that observed with the TCAs, and the potential for once daily administration.[5] Concurrent with these events have been significant structural (e.g. pharmaceutical formularies) and regulatory (e.g. required pharmacoeconomic evaluations) changes in the delivery, financing, and oversight of healthcare programmes throughout the world.[3,5] International cost-containment initiatives are increasingly mandating a demonstration of *value for money*, defined in terms of a measurable health and/or financial outcome and, in the case of medicines, attributable to a given expenditure, for a given pharmacotherapeutic option.[5]

Economic outcome assessment

Since 1990, researchers have employed five distinct methodological techniques to assess economic outcomes associated with the use of antidepressant pharmacotherapy:

- randomised controlled trials;
- meta-analyses stemming from the results of controlled clinical trials;
- decision-analytical models predicated on results stemming from randomised clinical trials and/or meta-analyses;
- retrospective data archive investigations;
- and prospective randomised naturalistic inquiry.

Herein the inherent strengths and weaknesses of each approach are considered, as is the effect of patient-level experience with antidepressant pharmacotherapy (i.e. access to medicines) on our understanding of the potential benefit(s) of a given pharmacotherapeutic option in the context of clinical practice.

Randomised controlled trials

The ecology of randomised controlled trials (RCTs) and their inherent utility and limitations were first addressed in earnest by White *et al.* in 1961.[6] RCTs are designed with the expressed intent of discerning information relative to the safety and efficacy of medicines, and thereby may not prove to be a suitable environment for answering questions regarding the effectiveness of a given compound.[7] The efficacy versus effectiveness quandary can be framed in terms of a trade-off between internal and external validity.[7] The RCT design yields enhanced internal validity, thereby affording causal inference regarding a given medicine and a given clinical or economic outcome. However, results stemming from RCTs have reduced external validity (i.e. generalisability) due to the very design structure and protocol requirements, which afford causal inference.[6] To date, RCTs incorporating the economic appraisal of antidepressant pharmacotherapy have not discerned significant differences between alternatives.[7]

Meta-analyses

Individual RCTs may not afford access to a sufficient sample size, and thereby power, to detect a significant difference in an outcome of interest across treatment arms (e.g. health service utilisation). Since 1993, four major meta-analyses have been conducted in an effort to compare outcomes stemming from RCTs examining TCAs and SSRIs. The first inquiry examined data from 63 RCTs and discerned no significant difference in terms of efficacy or discontinuation rate between TCAs and SSRIs.[8] A subsequent investigation questioned these findings, as the previous study had included 12 studies of heterocyclic antidepressants. Montgomery et al. included 42 published RCTs comparing SSRIs with TCAs and discerned a pooled discontinuation rate due to side effects of 14.9% for patients receiving an SSRI, and 19% among individuals receiving a TCA ($p \leq 0.01$).[9] In the seven placebo-controlled studies examined, the pooled discontinuation rate due to side effects for SSRIs was 19.0%, and 27.0% for patients receiving a TCA ($p \leq 0.01$). It was concluded that the risk–benefit calculation favoured the SSRIs as there were similar levels of efficacy, but significantly higher rates of discontinuation due to side effects with the TCAs. A third analysis by the same researchers extended the number of RCTs to 67 and discerned similar results.[10] However, in neither the second nor third meta-analysis were total discontinuation rates compared. The fourth effort examined overall discontinuation rates in 62 RCTs and discerned a modest, but statistically significant ($p \leq 0.05$) advantage for the SSRIs.[11]

The above findings have been used to support and refute a cost-minimisation perspective relative to antidepressant pharmacotherapy. However, as previously noted, results stemming from RCTs and meta-analyses may not equate with findings, and subsequent consequences, as seen in clinical practice. Therefore, in an effort to confront the external validity dilemma associated with results stemming from RCTs, and to assess the impact of said data on patients' well-being and health service

145

utilisation, modelling techniques have been employed in an effort to evaluate the cost-effectiveness of pharmaceuticals.[7]

Decision-analytical models

Decision-analytical modelling (DAM) affords a structured process for contrasting the costs and consequences associated with a new pharmacotherapeutic option relative to those of the current standard. However, the use of DAMs requires tolerance of uncertainty relative to some variables, the ability to represent complex relationships between inputs and outcomes accurately, an awareness of all factors that may influence said relationships, and thereby results, and a willingness to validate the accuracy of findings to the extent that validation is feasible.[12] Sensitivity analysis provides a robust mechanism by which to vary information of interest (inputs) within DAMs and subsequently assess the impact of said variation on findings (outcomes). The principal disadvantage associated with DAMs is that findings are predicated on the generalisability of data stemming from RCTs – an artificial environment far different from that of clinical practice.[7,12]

To date, publications utilising DAMs have employed data solely derived from RCTs, have estimated all requisite inputs, or have combined findings from RCTs with clinical and financial assumptions.[7,12] These efforts suffer from a variety of recurring shortcomings including concerns as to the soundness of model assumptions, the scope of inquiry, information inclusion and exclusion criteria, and the use of consensus panels.[7,12]

Retrospective database analyses

The fundamental threat to the validity of findings derived from DAMs is the extent to which basic assumptions and information stemming from RCTs accurately portray events in clinical practice.[7,12] Retrospective database research has attempted to overcome this limitation. Insurance company databases, originally designed for the adjudication and processing of patient-level medical claims, now often provide a rich source of population-based information regarding the utilisation of health services and/or clinical outcomes. However, the primary threat to the validity of outcomes stemming from database research is the potential for patient selection bias due to the non-random assignment of treatment options.

The first study to identify the economic consequences of subtherapeutic dosing with TCAs utilised data from the California Medicaid Program.[13] While data stemming from RCTs with TCAs suggests a treatment success rate of between 65 and 80%, only 20–25% of patients defined as having a major depressive disorder were found to have achieved a consistent, minimum therapeutic dose (defined daily dose), for a timeframe of six months or more. Treatment failure, defined as not having achieved a consistent, minimum therapeutic dose, for a timeframe of six months was associated with an increase in health service expenditures of over $1 000 per patient in the first year after initiating antidepressant pharmacotherapy.

A series of retrospective evaluations conducted in a network-model Health Maintenance Organisation (HMO) examined patterns of health service utilisation among patients diagnosed with single-episodic depression and prescribed either a TCA or an SSRI.[14,15] Patients prescribed an SSRI were consistently shown to accrue significantly lower ($p \leq 0.05$) health service expenditures (net of pharmacotherapy) relative to beneficiaries prescribed a TCA.

A retrospective intent-to-treat analysis utilised data from an HMO to contrast financial expenditure patterns stemming from receipt of an SSRI or a TCA.[16] Cohort assignment was based on initial receipt of either amitriptyline, fluoxetine, or nortriptyline for the treatment of single-episodic depression. Patients prescribed amitriptyline were over three times more likely to require a change in antidepressant pharmacotherapy (odds ratio, OR = 3.27, 95% confidence interval, CI = 2.31–5.49), while patients prescribed nortriptyline were nearly four times more likely to require a change in medication (OR = 3.82, 95% CI = 2.74–6.83) relative to patients initially prescribed fluoxetine. Consistent with the intent-to-treat design, all accrued health service expenditures were assigned to the pharmacotherapeutic option initially prescribed. Multivariate analyses revealed that initiation of antidepressant pharmacotherapy with amitriptyline resulted in a 25.7% increase in per capita depression-related health service expenditures per year, while initiation of antidepressant pharmacotherapy with nortriptyline resulted in a 28.1% increase in per capita depression-related health service expenditures per year relative to patients initially prescribed fluoxetine. A financial break-even point was achieved at the conclusion of month five, at which time all three intent-to-treat cohorts had comparable health service expenditures in total.

In a unique investigation, data from a private US health insurance programme were used to classify beneficiaries in accordance with their observed pattern of antidepressant use: early discontinuation; switching/augmentation; upward titration; partial compliance; and three-month use.[17] Overall costs of medical care were highest for patients in the switching/augmentation cohort ($7590) and early discontinuation cohort ($5610), and lowest for those in the upward titration, partial compliance, and three-month use cohorts ($3822, $4479, and $3393, respectively) ($p \leq 0.001$).

The utilisation patterns outlined above suggest that sensitivity analyses employed in DAMs would not, in the vast majority of instances, have accounted for the extent of the discrepancy between results stemming from RCTs and outcomes derived from database inquiries.[7,12] Therefore, findings stemming

147

from DAMs, based in large measure on meta-analyses of RCTs, are at best a starting point for assessing economic outcomes stemming from the use of antidepressant pharmacotherapy. Database research, while non-randomised, and thereby potentially subject to patient selection bias, affords insight into the pattern of health service utilisation and expenditures in clinical practice.

Prospective naturalistic inquiry

Decision-makers must weigh issues of safety, efficacy, and effectiveness when selecting among competing pharmacotherapeutic alternatives. To date, only one prospective study has been undertaken with the expressed intent of discerning the safety, efficacy, and effectiveness of antidepressant pharmacotherapy. In a randomised intent-to-treat analysis patients were prescribed either a TCA (desipramine or imipramine), or the SSRI fluoxetine.[18] At six months' post-initiation of pharmacotherapy, patients assigned to fluoxetine reported fewer adverse effects ($p \leq 0.05$), exhibited greater regimen duration ($p \leq 0.05$), were more often prescribed an adequate dose ($p \leq 0.05$), and were far less likely to require a change in pharmacotherapy ($p \leq 0.05$). Health service expenditures were comparable among the three cohorts at six months, with the greater procurement cost of fluoxetine offset by reductions in hospital and physician services. The naturalistic character of the intent-to-treat design yielded similar results to that obtained from retrospective database reviews.

Access to antidepressant pharmacotherapy

Experience with antidepressant pharmacotherapy within the context of clinical practice is requisite to understanding the benefit(s) of a given pharmacotherapeutic option. Recent studies suggest that access to antidepressant pharmacotherapy is influenced by a variety of factors, including the nature of the physician–patient relationship (e.g. initial encounter or follow up; length of encounter; physician specialty), patient expectations as regards the disease state and pharmacotherapy, patient characteristics such as age, gender, and race, and the wider social context in which the physician–patient encounter occurs, inclusive of the effect of pharmaceutical advertising and the financial incentives or disincentives intrinsic in a given health insurance programme.[19,20]

Future directions

The increasing prevalence of major depressive disorders and their associated morbidity, mortality, and economic consequence to the individual, society and the healthcare delivery system mandate the selection of safe, efficacious and effective treatment. Since 1990, the five study designs outlined above have been employed in efforts to discern and contrast financial outcomes stemming from the use of antidepressant pharmacotherapy. The selection of a given format reflects the objective(s) of a given inquiry, accessibility to quality data, and the time horizon in which the analysis was to have been conducted (phase III RCTs; postmarketing).

What emerges is the necessity of establishing a *portfolio* of evidence as to the safety, efficacy, and effectiveness of a given pharmacotherapeutic category (e.g. SSRIs) and/or a specific medication. As the case of antidepressants illustrates, the economic appraisal of pharmacotherapy requires an *iterative process* extending from the developmental (RCTs; meta-analyses; DAMs) through postmarketing phase (naturalistic inquiry; database reviews). Database reviews, while non-randomised, and prospective naturalistic inquiry appear to afford greater insight into the patterns of use and financial merits of prescribing specific pharmacotherapeutic options for the treatment of depression within the context of clinical practice as compared with RCTs, meta-analyses and DAMs. The portfolio of evidence to date suggests that the first-line use of SSRIs in the treatment of depression is clinically warranted and represents value for money.

References

1. Johnson J, Weissman MM, Klerman GL. Service utilization and social morbidity associated with depressive symptoms in the community. *JAMA* 1992;**267**:1478–83.
2. Blazer DG, Kessler RC, McGonagle KA, Swartz MS. The prevalence and distribution of major depression in a national community sample: the National Comorbidity Survey. *Am J Psychiatry* 1994;**151**:979–86.
3. Greenberg PE, Stiglin LE, Finkelstein SN, Berndt ER. The economic burden of depression in 1990. *J Clin Psychiatry* 1993;**54**: 405–18.
4. Murray CJL, Lopez AD, eds. *The Global Burden of Disease.* Cambridge, MA: Harvard University Press, 1996.
5. Sclar DA, Robinson LM, Skaer TL, Galin RS. Trends in the prescribing of antidepressant pharmacotherapy: office-based visits 1990–1995. *Clin Ther* 1998;**20**:871–84.
6. White KL, Williams TF, Greenberg BG. The ecology of medical care. *N Engl J Med* 1961;**265**:885–92.
7. Revicki DA, Frank L. Pharmacoeconomic evaluation in the real world. Effectiveness versus efficacy studies. *Pharmacoeconomics* 1999;**15**:423–34.
8. Song F, Freemantle N, Sheldon TA *et al.* Selective serotonin reuptake inhibitors: meta-analysis of efficacy and acceptability. *BMJ* 1993;**306**:683–7.
9. Montgomery SA, Henry J, McDonald G *et al.* Selective serotonin reuptake inhibitors: meta-analysis of discontinuation rates. *Int Clin Psychopharmacol* 1994;**9**:47–53.
10. Montgomery SA, Kasper S. Comparison of compliance between serotonin reuptake inhibitors and tricyclic antidepressants: a meta analysis. *Int Clin Psychopharmacol* 1995;**9** (Suppl 4):33–40.
11. Anderson IM, Tomenson BM. Treatment discontinuation with selective serotonin reuptake inhibitors compared with tricyclic antidepressants: a meta-analysis. *BMJ* 1995;**310**:1433–8.
12. Dolan JG. Can decision analysis adequately represent clinical problems? *J Clin Epidemiol* 1990;**43**:277–84.
13. McCombs JS, Nichol MB, Stimmel GE *et al.* The cost of antidepressant drug therapy failure: a study of antidepressant use patterns in a Medicaid population. *J Clin Psychiatry* 1990;**51** (Suppl 6):60–9.
14. Sclar DA, Robison LM, Skaer TL, *et al.* Antidepressant pharmacotherapy: economic

outcomes in a health maintenance organization. *Clin Ther* 1994;**16**:715–30.
15. Skaer TL, Sclar DA, Robison LM *et al.* Economic valuation of amitriptyline, desipramine, nortriptyline, and sertraline in the management of patients with depression. *Curr Ther Res Clin Exp* 1995;**56**:556–67.
16. Sclar DA, Skaer TL, Robison LM *et al.* Economic outcomes with antidepressant pharmacotherapy: a retrospective intent-to-treat analysis. *J Clin Psychiatry* 1998;**59** (Suppl 2):13–7.
17. Thompson D, Buesching D, Gregor KJ, Oster G. Patterns of antidepressant use and their relation to costs of care. *Am J Manag Care* 1996;**2**:1239–46.
18. Simon GE, VonKorff M, Heiligenstein JH *et al.* Initial antidepressant choice in primary care. Effectiveness and cost of fluoxetine vs tricyclic antidepressants. *JAMA* 1996;**275**:1897–1902.
19. Sclar DA, Robison LM, Skaer TL, Galin RS. What factors influence the prescribing of antidepressant pharmacotherapy? An assessment of national office-based encounters. *Int J Psychiatry Med* 1998;**28**:407–19.
20. Sclar DA, Robison LM, Skaer TL, Galin RS. Ethnicity and the prescribing of antidepressant pharmacotherapy: 1992–1995. *Harv Rev Psychiatry* 1999;**7**:29–36.

Antidepressant use in primary care

JOHN DONOGHUE

Introduction

There is good evidence from controlled studies that the older tricyclic antidepressants (TCAs) have efficacy at least as good as that of the newer selective serotonin-reuptake inhibitors (SSRIs).[1-3] However, for this potential for efficacy to be realised, clinicians must use these medicines effectively when treating patients.[4] Patients need to take an antidepressant at an effective dose for long enough for it to make a difference to the course of their illness.[4,5] In the United Kingdom, National Consensus Guidelines have advised that, to be effective, antidepressant treatment should continue for at least four months, and that for TCAs, the minimum effective dose is 125 mg/day of amitriptyline or its equivalent.[5] It is in this dimension of naturalistic use that TCAs have disadvantages compared with SSRIs.[6] The evidence that TCAs have been used suboptimally for many years, irrespective of the country and system of healthcare in which they have been used, is overwhelming. In contrast, patients treated with SSRIs are much more likely to receive effective treatment.[6]

Suboptimal use of antidepressants in primary care

Reports of suboptimal use of antidepressants for major depression have been appearing in the literature for the past quarter century.[6] In 1973 in the United Kingdom, Johnson found that patients prescribed antidepressants dropped out of treatment at an alarming rate: 68% of patients had stopped their antidepressant within four weeks.[7] In the same year, Kotin et al. in the United States reported that only 16% of depressed

151

patients admitted to hospital for treatment of depression had received at least 150 mg/day of imipramine or its equivalent before admission; over half had received no treatment at all.[8] Since then, similar findings have appeared all too frequently.[6]

In 1981, Johnson again investigated antidepressant use in primary care and found that only 25% of patients treated with a TCA received a dose above 75 mg/day.[9] The following year, a large multicentre study in the United States found that only 3% of depressed patients treated with an antidepressant received an antidepressant at an adequate dose for four weeks.[10] In 1982, Jick et al. in a study of nearly 7000 patients prescribed an antidepressant, found that 77% were prescribed less than 100 mg/day of TCA.[11]

In the 1990s, the availability of computerised medical record databases has enabled studies to take place in very large populations.[12–20] The first of these large studies to be published, a random retrospective database analysis of antidepressant use in the California Medicaid Program, found that, at best, only 20–25% of patients with major depressive disorder achieved a minimum therapeutic dose (defined as 75 mg/day of imipramine or its equivalent) for a minimum period of six months.[12] In Europe, studies include an investigation of how antidepressants were prescribed in Denmark, in a population of about 460 000 people: both the average doses and the most commonly prescribed doses of TCAs were below levels known to be effective in the treatment of depression.[13] In 1996, data from the United Kingdom became available from two studies that made use of a national medical records database of about 800 000 patient records,[14,15] and one that used a database covering a population of about 400 000 people in the Tayside district of Scotland.[16] In 1993 an analysis of over 100 000 prescriptions for antidepressants in patients with a diagnosis of depression[15] found average doses for older antidepressants to be: amitriptyline 55 mg/day; clomipramine 64 mg/day and dothiepin 76 mg/day. In 1995 average doses had changed marginally to: amitriptyline 59 mg/day; clomipramine 59 mg/day and dothiepin 77 mg/day.[15] The study in Scotland, in an analysis of over 85 000 prescriptions issued to more than 20 000 patients, found that at least 72% of patients prescribed a TCA received only a subtherapeutic dose, and 68% of patients took their antidepressant for less than 90 days.[16] These studies confirmed the findings from previous, smaller studies: that antidepressant use was suboptimal; that the majority of prescriptions for TCAs were in doses that had not been shown to be effective[12–16]; that patients were not taking antidepressants long enough for them to make a difference to the course of their illness[16]; and that there was little evidence of improvement over time.[15] These studies also found differences between the older TCAs and SSRIs: nearly 100% of patients treated with an SSRI received an effective dose.[14,15]

Similar findings have been made across Europe. In Sweden, average daily doses for amitriptyline and clomipramine were found to be 61 mg and 70 mg respectively.[17] A study of over 2500 patients in the Netherlands found that the mean daily dose of amitriptyline was 50 mg, and that most patients received less than four months' therapy.[18] In France, only 26% of primary care patients treated with a TCA received an effective dose,[21] and in Finland, 71% of patients prescribed a TCA received a dose below 75 mg/day.[22]

To date, the main focus has been on the suboptimal use of TCAs. However, there is an acute need to scrutinise the use of SSRIs. Although patients prescribed SSRIs nearly always receive an effective dose, still only one-third of patients complete four months of continuous therapy – the minimum recommended in most treatment guidelines.[19] There is clearly no room for complacency when prescribing these agents.

Few studies have compared TCAs and SSRIs using the parameters of both dose and length of treatment. Recently, a longitudinal study took place of antidepressant use in over 16 000 depressed patients in primary care in the United Kingdom starting treatment for a new episode of depression.[20] The findings were that less than 3% of patients who initiated treatment with a TCA (amitriptyline, dothiepin or imipramine) completed an adequate episode of treatment (four months' continuous treatment at an adequate dose – the minimum recommended in the United Kingdom National Consensus Guidelines), and those who initiated treatment with an SSRI (fluoxetine, paroxetine or sertraline) were 17 times more likely to complete an adequate episode of treatment.[20]

Alternative views

The findings that the use of TCAs is suboptimal have been questioned.[23-27] Clinical trials for antidepressants have been criticised, and their generalisability, particularly to primary care settings, called into doubt.[28] Opinions have been expressed that depression encountered in primary care is less severe than that seen in clinical trials, and responds to lower doses of antidepressant.[23-27] However, there seems to be little, if any objective evidence to support such views.[6]

One study that appears to lend some credence to these views is a recent meta-analysis of effectiveness of antidepressants by Bollini et al.[29] However, its conclusions should be viewed with extreme caution. There are several important limitations to the study. The first is the size and make-up of the dataset. The main controversy over antidepressant doses involves the prescribing of low dose TCAs in primary care settings.[13-18,21-23,25-27] Despite the very loose inclusion criteria that trials with as few as five patients per treatment arm, and as short a study period as three weeks, could be considered for inclusion in the meta-analysis, still only three studies involving TCAs were included. To make sweeping generalisations about the efficacy and tolerability of TCAs on the basis of only three studies seems at the least questionable. In addition, the average daily therapeutic doses of some of the study antidepressants and the conversion factors to an equivalent dose of imipramine are doubtful: the suggestion that at an equivalent dose of 100 mg/day of imipramine, fluoxetine and paroxetine at 20 mg/day are subtherapeutic is not supported by any evidence of which I am aware. The results use a therapeutic threshold of 100 mg/day of imipramine above which doses are regarded as being therapeutic and suggesting a trade-off between slightly reduced efficacy at this dose and tolerability. However, population-based studies consistently find that patients treated with TCAs are treated at doses significantly below this level.[6,8,10–18,20–23] The study ultimately fails to provide the answer to the question of whether the kinds of doses of TCAs used in primary care are effective. Yet the authors still make the assertion that prescribing a low dose of tricyclic seems to be a reasonable choice. This is untenable and may contribute to the perpetuation of this practice. Any differences in outcomes between high- and low-dose tricyclics are likely to be obscured by the small number of studies of TCAs, the inclusion of other antidepressants and the inaccurate computation of what constitutes an effective dose and how these doses may be converted to equivalent doses of imipramine. A recent study that investigated outcomes of such use of antidepressants found that over 60% of patients had moderate to severe major depression.[30] Similar findings have been made by other studies conducted in primary care settings: depressed patients fail to respond to low doses, and patients who are compliant with low-dose therapy often continue with their treatment unchanged despite a failure to respond.[30–34]

Conclusion

It seems reasonable to suggest that antidepressant use could be improved through education: there is little doubt that doctors need more training in the treatment of depression, and that patients need more and better information about antidepressant treatment. However, there is little evidence that this is actually happening.[6,15] What may help is clear, unequivocal, guidance on the crucial importance of depressed patients receiving an effective dose of antidepressant for long enough for it to change the course of their illness. Clinical governance requires that patients receive safe treatments of proven efficacy delivered effectively. There is little point in clinging to treatments that, despite evidence for their efficacy, are rarely used effectively. One suggestion may be to reserve TCAs for use by specialists. A continued emphasis on the primacy of the use of TCAs in primary care seems likely to perpetuate inadequate treatment[6,14,15,20] and poor outcomes,[30–35] with the prospect of failure of treatment, increased risk of developing chronic depression,[36,37] and possibly an increased risk of suicide[38].

References

1. Song F, Freemantle N, Sheldon T et al. Selective serotonin reuptake inhibitors: meta-analysis of efficacy and acceptability. BMJ 1993;306:683–7
2. Anderson IM, Tomenson BM. The efficacy of selective serotonin reuptake inhibitors in depression: a meta-analysis of studies against tricyclic antidepressants. J Psychopharmacol 1994;8:238–49
3. Hotopf M, Lewis G, Normand C. Are SSRIs a cost effective alternative to tricyclics? Br J Psychiatry 1996;168:404–9.
4. Potter WZ, Rudorfer MV, Monji H. The pharmacologic treatment of depression. N Eng J Med 1991;325:633–42.
5. Paykel ES, Priest RG. Recognition and management of depression in general practice: consensus statement BMJ 1992;305:1198–202.
6. Donoghue JM. Sub-optimal use of tricyclic antidepressants in primary care. [Editorial]. Acta Psychiatr Scand 1998;98:429–31.
7. Johnson DAW. Treatment of depression in general practice. BMJ 1973;1:18–20.
8. Kotin J, Post RM, Goodwin FK. Drug treatment of depressed patients referred for hospitalisation. Am J Psychiatry 1973;130:1139–41.
9. Johnson DAW. Depression: treatment compliance in general practice. Acta Psychiatr Scand 1981;63(Suppl 290):447–53.
10. Keller MB, Klerman GL, Lavori PW et al. Treatment received by depressed patients. JAMA 1982;248:1848–55.
11. Jick H, Dinan BJ, Hunter JW et al. Tricyclic antidepressants and convulsions. J of Clin Psychopharmacol 1983;3:182–5.
12. McCombs JS, Nichol MB, Stimmel GL et al. The cost of antidepressant drug therapy failure: a study of antidepressant use patterns in a Medicaid population. J Clin Psychiatry 1990;51 (6 Suppl):60–9.
13. Rosholm J–U, Hallas J, Gram LF. Outpatient utilisation of antidepressants: a prescription database analysis. J Affect Disord 1993;27:21–28.
14. Donoghue JM, Tylee A. The treatment of depression: prescribing patterns of antidepressants in primary care in the United Kingdom. Br J Psychiatry 1996;168:164–168.
15. Donoghue JM, Tylee A, Wildgust HJ. Cross sectional database analysis of antidepressant prescribing in general practice in the United Kingdom, 1993–5. BMJ 1996;313:861–2.
16. MacDonald TM, McMahon AD, Reid IC et al. Antidepressant drug use in primary care: a record linkage study in Tayside, Scotland. BMJ 1996;313:860–1.
17. Bingefors K, Isacson D, Von Knorring L. Antidepressant dose patterns in Swedish clinical practice. Int Clin Psychopharmacol 1997;12:283–290.
18. Gregor KJ, Hylan TR, Van Dijk PCM et al. Outpatient antidepressant utilisation in a Dutch sick fund. Am J Manag Care 1998;4:1150–60.
19. Donoghue J.M. Selective serotonin re–uptake inhibitor use in primary care: a five year naturalistic study Clin Drug Invest 1998;16:453–462
20. Dunn RL, Donoghue JM, Ozminkowski RJ et al. Longitudinal patterns of antidepressant prescribing in primary care in the United Kingdom: comparison with treatment guidelines. J Psychopharmacol 1999;13:136–143.
21. Rouillon F, Blachier C, Dreyfus JP et al. Etude pharmaco–épidémiologique de la consommation des antidepresseurs en population générale. L'encephale Sp 1996;1:39–48.
22. Isometsa E, Seppala I, Henriksson M et al. Inadequate dosaging in general practice of tricyclic vs. other antidepressants for depression Acta Psychiatr Scand 1998;98:451–4.
23. Thompson C, Thompson CM. The prescription of antidepressants in general practice: I. A critical review. Human Psychopharmacol 1989;4:91–102.
24. Kendrick, T. Prescribing antidepressants in general practice. [Editorial]. BMJ 1996;313:829–30.
25. Fish D. What is an effective dose? [letter]. BMJ 1997;314:826.
26. Moore MV. More on what is an effective dose. [letter]. BMJ 1997;314:826.
27. Tan RS. Low dose tricyclic antidepressants are effective in treating major depression. [letter] BMJ 1997;314:827.
28. Hotopf M, Lewis G, Normand C. Putting trials on trial – the costs and consequences of small trials in depression: a systematic review of methodology. J Epidemiol Community Health 1997;51:354–8.

29. Bollini P, Pampallona S, Tibaldi G *et al*. Effectiveness of antidepressants. Meta–analysis of dose–effect relationships in randomised clinical trials. *Br J Psychiatry* 1999;**174**:297–303.

30. Ali IM. Long–term treatment with antidepressants in primary care. *Psychiatric Bull* 1998;**22**:15–19.

31. Jones L, Simpson D, Brown AC et al. Prescribing psychotropic drugs in general practice: three year study. *BMJ* 1984;**289**:1045–8.

32. Goethe JW, Szarek BL, Cook WL. A comparison of adequately vs inadequately treated depressed patients. *J Nervous Mental Dis* 1988;**176**:465–70.

33. Paykel ES, Hollyman JA, Freeling P, Sedgwick P. Predictors of therapeutic benefit from amitriptyline in mild depression: a general practice placebo–controlled trial. *J Affect Disord* 1988;**14**:83–95.

34. Thompson C, Thompson CM. Prescribing of antidepressants in general practice. II. A placebo controlled trial of low dose dothiepin. *Human Psychopharmacol* 1989;**4**:191–204.

35. Brugha TS. Depression undertreatment: lost cohorts, lost opportunities? *Psycholog Med* 1995;**25**:3–6.

36. Keller MB, Lavori PW, Klerman GL *et al*. The persistent risk of chronicity in recurrent episodes of non–bipolar major depressive disorder: a prospective follow–up. *Am J Psychiatry* 1986;**143**:24–28.

37. Scott J, Barker WA, Eccleston D. The Newcastle Chronic Depression Study: patient characteristics and factors associated with chronicity. *Br J Psychiatry* 1988;**152**:28–33.

38. Isacsson G, Holmgren P, Wassermen D, Bergman U. Use of antidepressants among people committing suicide in Sweden. *BMJ* 1994;**308**:506–9.

THE DEBATE

The Motion

'This House believes that the new generation antidepressants are the most effective first-line treatment for depression.'

Chairman	DAVID HEALY MD
Debaters	
For the motion	JOHN DONOGHUE BSc MRPHARMS
	YVES LECRUBIER MD
Against the motion	JOHN GEDDES MD
	ALLAN HOUSE MD

Debate chairman's opening remarks

In this section we are going to debate the issue of new and old drugs for people who are depressed. But first I have to make an important disclaimer. The primary aim of this debate is to provide you with the most up-to-date unbiased published evidence, for and against the motion, to assist your own decision-making process. I do intend to take a vote at the end of the debate. However, as will become apparent, the result of that vote will not necessarily be the official view of the World Health Organization or any of the co-organizers. For that you should consult each organization separately.

The speakers have agreed that the new drugs are from Prozac onwards, although it has been pointed out that Prozac could be considered an old drug as it has been around for a long time! However for the conventions of this debate, it is a new drug. The new drugs are the SSRIs and post-SSRIs.

As you are aware, the old tricyclic antidepressant drugs are usually called TCAs these days. But there are drugs among the TCAs that are stronger serotonin-reuptake inhibitors than some drugs among the SSRI class, which are supposedly selective serotonin-reuptake inhibitors. The SSRIs, however, are not anymore generally selective than the TCAs were, except in so far as they have no actions on the noradrenaline system.

This debate will probably not cover the fact that, among the TCAs, there were drugs that were certainly lethal in overdose, and that is one reason for having other drugs. But neither are you going to hear that among the SSRIs, there is a considerable amount of evidence to suggest that one of

157

the best-selling induced suicide, probably at a rate of 1 per week over and above the rate that would have occurred in people who are depressed in primary care in the United Kingdom, if they had been left untreated.

So if the difference between the drugs is not in terms of their mode of action so much, or their risks, what is the difference? One difference, which you will not hear from our speakers between the TCAs and the SSRIs, is not any of these issues. The difference actually is patents. One group of drugs is on patent still and the other is not, and patents make corporations and corporations hire lawyers and lawyers advise what can be researched and what can be published. Now our debaters this afternoon have to pick their way through this, these are the gloves that they will have on them. There are things that they can talk to you about but there are also belts below which they cannot hit.

Finally, there is one further important issue. Fifty per cent of the audience here today is female, and when it comes to prescribing patterns, the gender of the prescriber is significant. Now I am sure you will hear during the debate, or certainly will hear tomorrow, that the SSRIs have greater compliance rates than the TCAs. It will be suggested to you that this is because they have got a better side-effect profile. In actual fact the greatest determinant of compliance is the relationship you have with your prescriber. In the United Kingdom, the people who prescribe SSRIs preferentially compared to the TCAs are female general practitioners. So are the compliance rates for SSRIs anything to do with the drugs or is it that women are just better therapists than men? This too will not be debated but I think it is worth bearing in mind, especially as our speakers today are all male!

Before commencing, I am going to ask you all to vote and vote again at the end on the motion that:

'This House believes that the new generation antidepressants are the most effective first-line treatment for depression.'

Can those of you who agree with the motion put your hands up.

- My estimate is about half of you voted in favour.
  You agree with the motion.

We will vote on this at the end; in between you have the men – they may not be able to treat depression but they can argue about it!

In favour of the motion:

First speaker: JOHN DONOGHUE

Despite a plethora of data from controlled clinical trials of antidepressants,[1-6] controversy remains over which class of antidepressants should generally be regarded as the optimal first-line choice for the majority of patients with major depression. Several approaches could be taken to address this question. These include:

- a systematic review of randomised, controlled trials;
- a review of the health economic data;
- and an understanding of how clinicians use these medicines in real-world clinical settings, particularly in primary care where the majority of cases of depression are treated.

Systematic reviews of controlled trials

Over the past decade there have been several meta-analyses of randomised controlled trials of antidepressants.[1-6] In comparisons mainly of tricyclic antidepressants (TCAs) with selective serotonin-reuptake inhibitors (SSRIs) they have found that efficacy is similar,[1-3] and that there are modest advantages in tolerability for the SSRIs.[4-6] Whether these modest advantages are clinically significant, or whether they justify the additional acquisition cost of the SSRIs is a question these studies are not able to answer.[3] Moreover, the generalisability of these findings to clinical practice is open to question.[7-8] Comparisons of tolerability in controlled trials have been based on drop-out rates.[1,4-6] However, studies where patient behaviour has been allowed to manifest itself freely have found large differences between the drop-out rates of TCAs and SSRIs – in favour of the SSRIs.[9,10] Thus an approach based solely on data from controlled trials does not give a satisfactory indication of which antidepressants are likely to be the most effective treatments in clinical practice.

Health economic evaluations

Similarly, health economic evaluations are inadequate to give clear guidance on this issue. Since clinical trials indicate that antidepressants such as the SSRIs have similar efficacy to the TCAs,[1-3] on an empirical level, using a cost-minimisation analysis, it may be assumed that the use of a more expensive drug with efficacy similar to existing medicines may increase the cost of treatment.[1,3-11] However, clinical trials alone may not provide sufficient information on which to base such assumptions.[3,9] Patients in clinical trials receive optimal care with the delivery of all treatments standardised to that of the most complex. In these circumstances, complex and demanding treatment regimens may perform better than they would in the practice setting, and cost differences between treatments will be hidden.[9] Moreover, in a short-term clinical trial that has been carried out to determine the efficacy and safety of the antidepressant, the endpoint will be a score on a depression rating scale that is unlikely to be a valid economic measure. Clinical practice will aim for longer-term treatment, as the endpoint is not merely reduction of the acute symptoms.[12]

A health economic approach can only answer this question if it is able to evaluate the impact of the drug on the totality of health expenditure. However, the system of healthcare in which the treatment is delivered may have an important influence on the total costs of care, resulting in the need to conduct separate health economic studies for each individual system of care.[9,13] Thus, although clinical trials are the gold standard for assessing the safety and efficacy of treatments under controlled conditions, and are an important influence on clinical practice, they provide little useful data that can be applied to considerations of cost effectiveness in clinical practice.[3] The application of cost-minimisation analyses to clinical trials of antidepressants is unlikely to be a valid pharmaco-economic measure.

Antidepressant use in clinical practice

Clinical trials have demonstrated that TCAs have efficacy at least as good as that of the newer SSRIs.[1-3] However, this is too narrow a perspective from which to evaluate how a drug will perform in delivering patient outcomes in real-world conditions.[14] Efficacy is a measure of the drug's ability to deliver an outcome under controlled and ideal conditions. However, for this potential for efficacy to be realised, clinicians must use these medicines optimally when treating patients. Effectiveness is a measure of the drug's performance in the real world where the drug is subject to variations in use resulting from the prescribing practice and follow-up care of physicians and the behaviour of patients. For treatment to be effective, patients must receive a therapeutic dose of antidepressant for a minimum of four months.[12] For tricyclic antidepressants, the minimum therapeutic dose is considered to be not less than 125 mg/day of amitriptyline or its equivalent.[12] It is in this dimension that the SSRIs prove to have significant advantages. There is overwhelming evidence that TCAs have been used suboptimally for many years, irrespective of the country and system of healthcare in which they have been used.[15] In contrast, there is robust evidence from very large studies that patients treated with SSRIs are more likely to receive effective treatment.[15-19]

However, findings that doses of tricyclic antidepressants used in clinical practice are inadequate are considered by some to be controversial. The design of clinical trials for antidepressants has been criticised, and their generalisability, particularly to primary care settings, may be limited.[7] Anecdotal evidence has been cited that the severity of depression encountered in primary care is different from that seen in clinical trials, and does not require to be treated with full doses of antidepressant.[20-24] However, there is little, if any, systematic evidence to support such views. Studies conducted in primary care settings have found consistently that depressed patients fail to respond to low doses, and that patients who are compliant with low-dose therapy continue with their treatment unchanged despite a failure to respond.[15]

A recent meta-analysis of effectiveness of antidepressants[25] suggested that a dose of 100 mg/day of TCA could be regarded as an effective dose, and that at this dose there may be a trade-off between efficacy and tolerability. However, population-based studies consistently find that most patients treated with TCAs receive doses significantly below this level.[16-20,26-40] Moreover, despite the very liberal inclusion criteria that trials with as few as five patients per treatment arm and as short a study period as three weeks could be considered for inclusion in the meta-analysis, still only three studies involving tricyclic antidepressants were included.[25] It seems unsafe to base such a wholesale generalisation about the efficacy and tolerability of TCAs on such a small number of studies.

A recent longitudinal study of over 16 000 depressed patients in primary care in the United Kingdom[19] was able to provide quantitative evidence of the difference in the treatment received by patients starting treatment with a TCA or SSRI. It found that less than 3% of patients who initiated treatment with a TCA completed an adequate episode of treatment (four months' continuous treatment at an adequate dose – the minimum recommended in the United Kingdom National Consensus Guidelines[12]), and those who initiated treatment with an SSRI were 17 times more likely to complete an adequate episode of treatment.

None of the three approaches to exploring the question of which antidepressants should be regarded as the best first-line option for the majority of patients is wholly satisfactory. Controlled trials are the best means of reducing bias, but the generalisability of their findings is open to question. Data from current health economic studies are insufficient to inform any decision for the National Health Service (NHS). Population-based studies are open to selection bias and a range of external influences on outcomes. However, a synthesis of the data from all of these approaches leads to several conclusions:

- TCAs and SSRIs have similar efficacy, with moderate tolerability advantages for the SSRIs.
- There are no unequivocal health economic data to suggest that in a NHS context either treatment is more cost-effective than the other.
- In clinical practice in primary care settings – where the majority of cases of depression are treated – TCAs are used suboptimally on a massive scale. Patients treated with an SSRI are much more likely to receive effective treatment.

The last conclusion is probably the most important. It would not matter if a TCA had better efficacy than an SSRI if, in clinical practice, the added complexity of treatment with a TCA resulted in the SSRI being the only one that was used effectively. Similarly, evidence of better cost-effectiveness for a TCA in a controlled study would be of little use if the SSRI was more likely to be used effectively in clinical practice, as is indeed the case. There can be little doubt that in a comparison between TCAs and SSRIs, the newer generation antidepressants offer the most effective first-line treatment of depression. They do not have superior efficacy; they are simply better tolerated and easier to use, and this results in their being used more effectively in real-world conditions.

Clinical governance demands that we provide safe and effective treatment to patients. There seems little point in clinging to treatments that, despite evidence for their efficacy, are rarely used effectively. A continued emphasis on the use of TCAs in primary care will perpetuate poor outcomes,[41] with the prospect of failure of treatment,[12,20,31,40] and possibly an increased risk of suicide.[42] As we enter the new millennium, SSRIs should be regarded as the first-line treatment for depression in primary care.

References

1. Song F, Freemantle N, Sheldon T *et al.* Selective serotonin reuptake inhibitors: meta-analysis of efficacy and acceptability. *BMJ* 1993;**306**:683–7.
2. Anderson IM, Tomenson BM. The efficacy of selective serotonin reuptake inhibitors in depression: a meta-analysis of studies against tricyclic antidepressants. *J Psychopharmacol* 1994;**8**:238–249.
3. Hotopf M, Lewis G, Normand C. Are SSRIs a cost effective alternative to tricyclics? *Br J Psychiatry* 1996;**168**:404–9.
4. Montgomery SA, Henry J, McDonald G, Dinan T *et al.* Selective serotonin reuptake inhibitors: meta-analysis of discontinuation rates. *Int Clin Psychopharmacol* 1994;**9**:47–53.
5. Anderson IM, Tomenson BM. Treatment discontinuation rates with selective serotonin reuptake inhibitors compared with tricyclic antidepressants: a meta-analysis. *BMJ* 1995;**310**:1433–8.
6. Hotopf M, Hardy R, Lewis G. Discontinuation rates of SSRIs and tricyclic antidepressants: a meta-analysis and investigation of heterogeneity. *Br J Psychiatry* 1997;**170**:120–7.
7. Hotopf M, Lewis G, Normand C. Putting trials on trial – the costs and consequences of small trials in depression: a systematic review of methodology. *J Epidemiol Community Health* 1997;**51**:354–358.
8. Simon G, Wagner E, Von Korff M. Cost-effectiveness comparisons using 'real world' randomised trials: the case of new antidepressant drugs. *J Clin Epidemiol* 1995;**48**:363-373
9. Simon GE, Von Korff M, Heiligenstein JH *et al.* Initial antidepressant choice in primary care. *JAMA* 1996;**275**:1897–1902.
10. Demyttenaere K, Van Ganse E, Gregoire J *et al.* Compliance in depressed patients treated with fluoxetine or amitriptyline. *Int Clin Psychopharmacol* 1998;**13**:11–17.
11. Freemantle N, Long A, Mason J, *et al.* The treatment of depression in primary care. *Effective Health Care Bull* 1993;**5**:1–12.
12. Paykel ES, Priest RG. Recognition and management of depression in general practice: consensus statement. *BMJ* 1992;**305**:1198–202.
13. Rosenbaum JF, Hylan TR. Costs of depressive disorders: a review. In: Maj M, Sartorius N, eds. *Evidence and Experience in Psychiatry, Volume 1: depressive disorders.* p.401–49, Chichester, John Wiley, 1999.
14. Reeder CE. Overview of pharmacoeconomics and pharmaceutical outcomes evaluations.

Am J Health-System Pharmacy 1995;**52**(Suppl 3):S5–8.

15. Donoghue JM. Sub-optimal use of tricyclic antidepressants in primary care [Editorial]. *Acta Psychiatr Scand* 1998;**98**:429–31.

16. Donoghue JM, Tylee A. The treatment of depression: prescribing patterns of antidepressants in primary care in the United Kingdom. *Br J Psychiatry* 1996;**168**:164–8.

17. Donoghue JM, Tylee A, Wildgust HJ. Cross sectional database analysis of antidepressant prescribing in general practice in the United Kingdom, 1993–5. *BMJ* 1996;**313**:861–2.

18. Donoghue J, Katona C, Tylee A. The treatment of depression: antidepressant prescribing for elderly patients in primary care. *Pharmaceut J* 1998;**260**:500–2.

19. Dunn RL, Donoghue JM, Ozminkowski RJ *et al.* Longitudinal patterns of antidepressant prescribing in primary care in the UK: comparison with treatment guidelines. *J Psychopharmacol* 1999;**13**(2):136–43.

20. Thompson C, Thompson CM. The prescription of antidepressants in general practice: I. A critical review. *Human Psychopharmacol* 1989;**4**:91–102.

21. Kendrick, T. Prescribing antidepressants in general practice. *BMJ* 1996;**313**:829–30.

22. Fish D. What is an effective dose? [letter]. *BMJ* 1997;**314**:826

23. Moore MV. More on what is an effective dose [letter]. *BMJ* 1997;**314**:826

24. Tan RS. Low dose tricyclic antidepressants are effective in treating major depression. [letter]. *BMJ* 1997;**314**:827.

25. Bollini P, Pampallona S, Tibaldi G *et al.* Effectiveness of antidepressants. Meta-analysis of dose–effect relationships in randomised clinical trials. *Br J Psychiatry* 1999;**174**:297–303.

26. Johnson DAW. Treatment of depression in general practice. *BMJ* 1973;**1**:18–20.

27. Kotin J, Post RM, Goodwin FK. Drug treatment of depressed patients referred for hospitalisation. *Am J Psychiatry* 1973;**130**:1139–41.

28. Keller MB, Klerman GL, Lavori PW *et al.* Treatment received by depressed patients. *JAMA* 1982;**248**:1848–55.

29. Jick H, Dinan BJ, Hunter JW *et al.* Tricyclic antidepressants and convulsions. *J Clin Psychopharmacol* 1983;**3**:182–5.

30. Jones L, Simpson D, Brown AC *et al.* Prescribing psychotropic drugs in general practice: three year study. *BMJ* 1984;**289**:1045–8.

31. McCombs JS, Nichol MB, Stimmel GL *et al.* The cost of antidepressant drug therapy failure: a study of antidepressant use patterns in a Medicaid population. *J Clin Psychiatry* 1990;**51**(6, Suppl):60–69.

32. Katon W, Von Korff M, Lin E *et al.* Adequacy and duration of antidepressant treatment in primary care. *Med Care* 1992;**30**:67–76.

33. Rosholm J-U, Hallas J, Gram LF. Outpatient utilisation of antidepressants: a prescription database analysis. *J Affect Disord* 1993;**27**:21–28.

34. Simon G, Von Korff M, Wagner EH, Barlow W. Patterns of antidepressant use in community practice. *Gen Hosp Psychiatry* 1993;**15**:399–408.

35. Arpino C, Da Cas R, Donini G *et al.* The use and misuse of antidepressant drugs in a random sample of the population of Rome, Italy. *Acta Psychiatr Scand* 1995;**92**:7–9.

36. Munizza C, Tibaldi G, Bollini P *et al.* Prescription pattern of antidepressants in out-patient psychiatric practice. *Psychol Med* 1995;**25**:771–8.

37. MacDonald TM, McMahon AD, Reid IC *et al.* Antidepressant drug use in primary care: a record linkage study in Tayside, Scotland. *BMJ* 1996;**313**:860–1.

38. Weiller E, Lecrubier Y, Boyer P. Antidepressant use in general practice. *Therapie* 1996;**51**:429–30.

39. Bingefors K, Isacson D, Von Knorring L. Antidepressant dose patterns in Swedish clinical practice. *Int Clin Psychopharmacol* 1997;**12**(5):283–90.

40. Ali IM. Long-term treatment with antidepressants in primary care. *Psychiatr Bull* 1998;**22**:15–9.

41. Brugha TS. Depression undertreatment: lost cohorts, lost opportunities? *Psychol Med* 1995;**25**:3–6.

42. Isacsson G, Holmgren P, Wassermen D, Bergman U. Use of antidepressants among people committing suicide in Sweden. *BMJ* 1994;**308**:506–9.

Second speaker: YVES LECRUBIER

It is generally accepted that long-term strategies for the identification and treatment of depression are of increasing importance as depression will become the second most disabling condition worldwide by the year 2020. Pharmacotherapy for depression has improved in recent years and this paper sets out to discuss the relative merits of the newer generation of antidepressants.

In order to evaluate the advantages of the new versus 'first generation' of antidepressants, selective serotonin-reuptake inhibitors (SSRIs), a prototypic example of the new antidepressant treatments, will be compared with the 'first generation' therapeutic agents for depression, tricyclic antidepressants (TCAs).

Development of the new antidepressant agents has progressed substantially during the last three decades due to three major factors:

- A greater understanding of the nature of the interaction between antidepressants and central neurobiological transmitter systems has allowed drugs to be developed that target specific components of the neurotransmitter system.
- More stringent requirements and methodology are now demanded by international regulatory authorities in order to demonstrate an acceptable risk/benefit ratio.
- An increasing importance has been given to management with an improved definition of an adequate dosing regimen and easier dosing schedule.

This paper will discuss the situation with the SSRIs and the TCAs against each of these three factors.

Specific neurobiological properties

The antidepressant efficacy of the TCAs has been linked to two neurobiological properties: (1) the inhibition of serotonin reuptake (as exemplified by clomipramine); and/or (2) the inhibition of noradrenaline reuptake (as exemplified by desipramine). SSRIs inhibit only serotonin reuptake[1] and while maintaining therapeutic efficacy demonstrate a considerably improved tolerability profile due to their reduced ability to interact with other neurotransmitter systems. Side effects commonly observed with SSRIs such as nausea or sexual dysfunction are linked to the serotonergic mechanism of action and are also reported with serotonergic TCAs (e.g. clomipramine). In contrast, more serious adverse events have been reported following TCA administration due to their ability to interact with components of cholinergic, adrenergic and histaminergic neuro-transmission:

164

- cognitive dysfunction, dry mouth, constipation, increased intraocular pressure and problems in patients with prostatitis (anticholinergic effects);
- orthostatic hypotension leading to falls and fractures (adrenergic blockade);[2]
- sedation and impairment of psychomotor performances (antihistaminic effects).[3]

The improved tolerability profile observed with the SSRIs may even be underestimated, as the currently favoured method of reporting the frequency of adverse events in a clinical trial does not allow for a consideration of their clinical impact and severity. This is justified for regulatory purposes but does not describe the reality of the side effect burden associated with TCA use. For example, 90% of patients in a clinical trial may report adverse events with TCAs compared with 70% in the placebo group; however, the clinical impact of the TCA-emergent adverse events may differ considerably from those associated with placebo.

A documented and controlled risk:benefit ratio

The adoption of screening procedures both at the preclinical level and in early clinical trials has resulted in the development of antidepressant agents with an improved safety profile compared with the TCAs. Unlike the TCAs, the SSRIs do not possess quinidine-like antiarrhythmic activity and this has reduced the risk of serious and potentially lethal cardiovascular toxicity.[4] There is a substantial reduction in the ability of the newer antidepressants to induce convulsions, and the effects on liver and renal functions are well studied and documented. Although interactions with different cytochrome P450s have been reported[5] for each agent in the SSRI class, these have proved to be of no major clinical relevance. The incidence of clinically relevant drug–drug interactions is very low with the exception of an interaction with drugs with a similar mechanism of action, i.e. those that increase serotonin levels. An index of the relevance of this improved safety profile is the much lower proportion of deaths after antidepressant overdose with SSRIs ($2.02/10^6$ prescriptions) compared with TCAs ($34.14/10^6$).[6]

At a clinical level, the efficacy of all new antidepressants is clearly superior to placebo. Furthermore, almost all controlled trials show similar efficacy for TCAs and SSRIs, which is as expected from drugs with a similar mechanism of action. These findings are confirmed in a recent meta-analysis[7] where the majority of trials comparing SSRIs and TCAs show minimal differences (Figure 7). The only exception is in hospitalised depressed patients where TCAs demonstrated some superiority.[7] In my opinion this is due to the convergence of three factors.

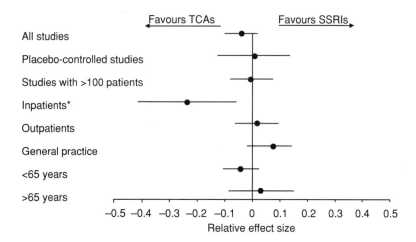

Figure 7 Meta-analysis of 102 randomised controlled trials (10 706 patients) *p=0.012.

1. It is not a TCA phenomenon in general, but related to clomipramine, which has displayed particular efficacy in this population. No dose-response data exist for clomipramine but the dose of 150 mg used in the trials is probably the equivalent of doses of more than 300 mg of imipramine. This explains why many clinicians with a long-term experience of clomipramine use 75–100 mg in Europe as a first-line dose.
2. The poor treatment compliance commonly observed with TCAs can be improved when nurses administer drugs to hospitalised patients who are often already familiar with the adverse event profile of these agents.
3. In clinical trials, concomitant treatment with hypnotics and anxiolytics is commonly prohibited. Patients receiving SSRIs lack this treatment whereas those receiving TCAs have the sedative property embodied in the molecule. Nevertheless, it is probably better to prescribe an independent sedative substance to hospitalised patients who require it.

All new antidepressant treatments must demonstrate long-term efficacy in clinical trials, e.g. acute treatment phase followed by a 6–12-month relapse prevention study. Of the first-generation antidepressants, only imipramine, desipramine and amitriptyline have convincing long-term data.[8–11]

Management issues

The management of antidepressant treatment has improved enormously with the new generation of antidepressants. The recommended starting dose for treatment is chosen according to the results of modern dose range-finding studies. A higher dose (usually twice) benefits only a minority of patients (due to the flat dose–effect curve). Because of the good tolerability profile of the SSRIs, the initial starting dose is suitable for the majority of patients with the possible exception of cases of initial severe nausea and, as with all antidepressants, in patients with a history of panic disorder where a lower starting dose may be recommended. With TCAs dose range-finding data were either never collected or impossible to determine, e.g. starting doses of imipramine range between 50 and 300 mg and tolerance may be poor even at 50 mg.

The pioneering work of Ayd[12] has demonstrated the improved treatment compliance that can be obtained with drugs requiring only a single daily dose; the majority of new antidepressants meet this criterion. The consequences of this improved management of treatment are dramatic in terms of mental healthcare and helps to explain the success of SSRIs in the primary care setting as shown in the following conservative example.

Final percentage of depressed patients benefiting from drug treatment:

TCAs: 70% responders, adequate dose 33%, compliance 30% ⇨ 7% benefit from treatment.

SSRIs: 60% responders, adequate dose 90%, compliance 66% ⇨ 35.5% benefit from treatment.

Even if a mildly better efficacy is assumed for the TCAs compared with the SSRIs (although this is not the author's view) the final effectiveness is still very largely in favour of the SSRIs. It is clear that a good tolerability and safety profile and the absence of major interactions with most other drugs also substantially simplify the use of SSRIs, in particular, in special populations such as the elderly.

False beliefs

'The cost of new antidepressants is higher than that of TCAs.'

This phenomenon is true for any new drug class (e.g. antihypertensives, antibiotics); however cost implications appear to be given greater importance in psychiatry. Nevertheless, the cost of drugs is relatively small in the overall treatment cost of depression. The improved compliance, reduced relapse rate after stopping medication, earlier return to work and life activities, the higher percentage of patients benefiting from the new drugs, and the improved safety profile, all largely compensate for the difference in drug price. A study in the United Kingdom[13] and also one conducted in the United States[14] have reported similar or even lower direct costs for depressed patients treated with an SSRI compared with a TCA.

'The size of the drug effect is small, inflating the cost of depression.'[15]

The experimental design of most clinical trial programmes is determined by the questions posed by regulatory authorities in order to demonstrate the efficacy of the new drug. However, the restrictions that this can place on the clinical trial design can have major implications on the trial results: placebo-controlled trials with a very high number of clinic visits (10–12 in 12 weeks) are known to inflate the response rate in the placebo group; the use of fixed dose is often recommended, usually from the beginning of treatment, thus not allowing treatment to be titrated according to the needs of the individual; no concomitant medication (hypnotics, anxiolytics) is allowed; an intent-to-treat analysis is conducted whereby the results of patients with an early drop-out are taken into account throughout the duration of a trial.

Furthermore, recruitment to clinical trials commonly excludes a majority of the depressed population (previous treatment, psychiatric comorbidity, physical illness) and, due to the inclusion of a placebo group, the most severely depressed and suicidal patients. These limitations prevent such clinical trials from providing a true indication of the magnitude of the drug effect.

Conclusions

Considering the more robust clinical data available for the newer antidepressants combined with a simpler dosing schedule and improved tolerability profile, one wonders if the question 'Are SSRIs better than TCAs?' should not be changed to the more relevant question 'What justifies the prescription of TCAs as a first-line treatment?' I would propose that only patients who have not responded to the newer antidepressant classes and who have a high motivation to take drugs with a poor tolerability profile and serious safety problems should be administered such treatment.

References

1. Leonard BE. Selective serotonin re-uptake inhibitors. The comparative pharmacological properties of selective serotonin re-uptake inhibitors in animals. In: Feighner JP and Boyer WP, eds. *Perspectives in Psychiatry*, 2nd edn. Volume 5, pp. 35–62. Chichester: John Wiley, 1996.
2. Glassman AH, Preud'homme XA. Review of the cardiovascular effects of heterocyclic antidepressants. *J Clin Psychiatry* 1993;**54** (Suppl):16–22.
3. Hindmarch I, Shamsi Z, Stanley N, Fairweather DB. A double-blind, placebo-controlled investigation of the effects of fexofenadine, loratadine and promethazine on cognitive and psychomotor function. *Br J Clin Pharmacol* 1999;**48**:200–6.
4. Roose SP, Laghrissi-Thode F, Kennedy JS *et al.* Comparison of paroxetine and nortriptyline in depressed patients with ischemic heart disease. *JAMA* 1998;**279**:287–91.
5. Brosen K, Rasmussen BB. Selective serotonin re-uptake inhibitors. Pharmacokinetics and drug interactions. In: Feighner JP and Boyer WP, eds. *Perspectives in Psychiatry*, 2nd edn. Volume 5, pp. 87–108. Chichester: John Wiley, 1996.
6. Henry JA. Epidemiology and relative toxicity of antidepressant drugs in overdose. *Drug Safety* 1997;**16**:374–90.

7. Anderson IM. Selective serotonin reuptake inhibitors versus tricyclic antidepressants: a meta-analysis of efficacy and tolerability. *J Affect Disord* (in press).
8. Prien RF, Kupfer DJ, Mansky PA *et al.* Drug therapy in the prevention of recurrences in unipolar and bipolar affective disorders. Report of the NIMH Collaborative Study Group comparing lithium carbonate, imipramine, and a lithium carbonate-imipramine combination. *Arch Gen Psychiatry* 1994;11:1096–104.
9. Frank E, Kupfer DJ. Three-year outcomes for maintenance therapies in recurrent depression. *Arch Gen Psychiatry* 1990;47:1093–9.
10. Kocsis JH, Friedman RA, Markowitz JC *et al.* Maintenance therapy for chronic depression. A controlled clinical trial of desipramine. *Arch Gen Psychiatry* 1996;53:769–74; discussion 775–6.
11. Montgomery SA, Reimitz PE, Kivkov M. Mirtazapine versus amitriptyline in the long-term treatment of depression: a double-blind placebo-controlled study. *Int Clin Psychopharmacol* 1998;13:63–73.
12. Ayd FJ Jr. Single daily dose of antidepressants. [Editorial.] *JAMA* 1974;230:263–4.
13. Jonsson B, Bebbington PE. What price depression? The cost of depression and the cost-effectiveness of pharmacological treatment. *Br J Psychiatry* 1994;164:665–73.
14. Bentkover JD, Feighner JP. Cost analysis of paroxetine versus imipramine in major depression. *Pharmacoeconomics* 1995;8:223–32.
15. Stewart A. Choosing an antidepressant: effectiveness based pharmacoeconomics. *J Affect Disord* 1998;48:125–33.

Against the motion

First speaker: JOHN GEDDES

It is reasonable to substitute a new treatment for an old if there is reliable evidence that either:

• the newer treatment is more effective than existing treatments;

or

• the newer treatment is better tolerated with fewer side effects than existing treatments

If the answer is yes to either question or both, then we also need to know if the advantage is clinically significant and, if so, whether the benefit is worth the acquisition costs.

It is generally assumed that the burden of proof for demonstrating the superiority of a new treatment lies with the proponent of the new treatment.[1] In the case of new drugs, this will usually be the drug company involved. The additional evidence requirements that are increasingly being requested by purchasers of healthcare is seen as a 'fourth step' to be negotiated by the industry and has initially led to some industry disquiet. The reasons for this include understandable industry concerns about adding to the already considerable development costs of new compounds and also that, in many cases, the quality of evidence required prior to introducing a new treatment will exceed that supporting the use of existing treatments.

Generally, it is both the main priority and also easier to obtain reliable answers to questions of efficacy and tolerability than of cost-effectiveness.

Therefore many of the most controversial decisions exist in the areas where there is little or unreliable evidence of clinically relevant benefit, but where the cost consequences of treatment decisions are substantial. One such case is the place of new antidepressants in clinical practice. Despite a continuing controversy about the place of the newer drugs in clinical practice, the use of newer drugs such as the selective serotonin-reuptake inhibitors (SSRIs) has increased dramatically over the past decade.[2]

Efficacy of antidepressants

We know that antidepressants are an effective treatment for depressive disorders.[3] There is general agreement, on the basis of several systematic reviews and meta-analyses, that the newer antidepressants are no more efficacious in the short-term than the older tricyclic drugs. The most recent Cochrane review of 98 randomised controlled trials included 5044 patients assigned to SSRIs and 4510 patients treated with older antidepressants.[4] This consensus about efficacy is of interest because all of these trials are industry-sponsored Phase 3 pivotal trials undertaken mainly for regulatory purposes, with a number of serious flaws (short duration, high drop-out rates, little use of intention-to-treat analysis, and outcome measures of uncertain clinical meaning).[5] Furthermore, despite the increasing recognition that depression is frequently a recurrent illness requiring maintenance drug treatment, there are few long-term trials of new drugs compared to either placebo or older drugs. It is possible that the real-world effects of antidepressants are different from those observed in these short-term trials. There are few examples of effectiveness trials in psychiatry – but Simon et al. have reported the long-term outcomes of a real-world comparison of a policy of using SSRIs as first line compared to tricyclic antidepressants (TCAs).[6] In this study, patients could change from one arm to another and many patients allocated to TCAs changed over to SSRIs early in the trial. Despite this, drug costs were substantially higher in the group that commenced with an SSRI although there was no difference in clinical outcome. Notably, the proportions of patients who continued taking an antidepressant long-term was similar in the groups and so it does not appear that the experience of early changeover led to long-term reluctance to continue treatment. Total healthcare costs were high with high variability, but there was no clear difference between groups.

Tolerability of antidepressants

Several meta-analyses and systematic reviews have demonstrated a statistically significant difference in drop-out rates in the short-term trials.[7-10] Anderson and Tomensen found the pooled risk ratio for drop-out to be 0.90 (95% confidence interval 0.84–0.97).[11] This indicates that there is a small, but statistically significant advantage in favour of the SSRIs in terms of relative drop-out. However, the pooled absolute rate of drop-out from these trials was 30.8% on SSRI compared to 33.4% on older drugs, an absolute difference of just 2.6%. Therefore, the relative advantage of SSRIs needs to be put into the context of a high overall drop-out rate from the trials. Of course, the validity of using drop-out from Phase 3 trials as an indicator of acceptability in real-world clinical practice is uncertain. The actual difference between the drugs may be greater or smaller. The small benefit in overall tolerability should be contrasted with the larger differences in specific adverse effects[12] (see Table 8). The data in the table are those reported in the short-term clinical trials and do not include other now well-recognised adverse effects of SSRIs such as sexual dysfunction. The adverse effects of newer drugs take time to become known. However, it is clear that the different drugs have very different side-effect profiles.

Table 8 Specific side effects of selective serotonin-reuptake inhibitors and tricyclic antidepressants (from Trindade and Menon[12])

Outcome	SSRI weighted event rate	TCA weighted event rate	Relative risk reduction (95% CI)	Weighted absolute risk reduction	Number needed to treat (95% CI)
Dry mouth	21%	55%	61% (54–66)	34%	3 (3–4)
Constipation	10%	22%	46% (33–56)	12%	9 (7–13)
Dizziness	13%	23%	45% (30–56)	10%	10 (8–16)
Nausea	22%	12%	83% (53–119)	10%	11 (8–15)
Diarrhoea	13%	5%	130% (17–355)	8%	13 (8–59)
Anxiety	13%	7%	77% (18–165)	6%	16 (10–53)
Agitation	14%	8%	66% (-9–195)	5%	19 (10–437)
Insomnia	12%	7%	60% (25–105)	4%	22 (15–46)
Nervousness	15%	11%	44% (9–91)	3%	29 (17–99)
Headache	17%	14%	31% (12–53)		33 (19–127)

Summary

Ultimately, decisions about when to use the SSRIs and newer antidepressants compared to the older drugs will depend on the funding agents' willingness to pay for a relative small and rather uncertain benefit in overall tolerability. Globally, relatively affluent healthcare systems are likely to pay for the newer drugs – especially in the face of high patient demand. Even then, purchasers will want to make sure that they are getting value for money. Over time, the relative acquisition costs of drugs fall, especially once the patent expires as it has recently in the case of fluoxetine. Drug companies will be keen to maximise sales of a new drug early on – though there may be limited evidence at that stage. In less affluent healthcare systems, where there is limited funding available, the older drugs are likely to be used because the extra costs may be more beneficially spent elsewhere. Even when a healthcare system can afford the newer antidepressants, it would be inappropriate to recommend that the newer drugs should always be used. Doctors should consider the different side-effect profiles and tailor the treatment according to the patient's preference and clinical need.

Ladies and gentlemen, I call upon you to vote against the motion.

References

1. Eddy DM. Clinical decision making: from theory to practice. Principles for making difficult decisions in difficult times. *JAMA* 1994;**271**:1792–8.
2. Eccles M, Freemantle N, Mason J, and North of England Guidelines Development Project. North of England Evidence-based Guideline Development Project: summary of guidelines for the choice of antidepressants for depression in primary care. *Family Practice* 1999;**16**:103–11.
3. Joffe R, Sokolov S, Streiner D. Antidepressant treatment of depression: a meta-analysis. *Can J Psychiatry* 1996;**41**:613–6.
4. Geddes JR, Freemantle N, Mason J et al. SSRIs versus alternative antidepressants in depressive disorder. In: Cochrane Collaboration. *Cochrane Library*. Oxford: Update Software, 1999.
5. Hotopf M, Lewis G, Normand C. Putting trials on trial – the costs and consequences of small trials in depression: a systematic review of methodology. *J Epidemiol Community Health* 1997;**51**:354–8.
6. Simon GE, Heiligenstein J, Revicki D et al. Long-term outcomes of initial antidepressant drug choice in a 'real world' randomized trial. *Arch Fam Med* 1999;**8**:319–25.
7. Song F, Freemantle N, Sheldon TA et al. Selective serotonin reuptake inhibitors: meta-analysis of efficacy and acceptability. *BMJ* 1993;**306**:683–7.
8. Montgomery SA, Kasper S. Comparison of compliance between serotonin reuptake inhibitors and tricyclic antidepressants: a meta-analysis. *Int Clin Psychopharmacol* 1995; **9**:(Suppl) 4:33–40.
9. Anderson IM, Tomenson BM. Treatment discontinuation with selective serotonin reuptake inhibitors compared with tricyclic antidepressants: a meta-analysis. *BMJ* 1995;**310**:1433–8.
10. Hotopf M, Hardy R, Lewis G. Discontinuation rates of SSRIs and tricyclic antidepressants: a meta-analysis and investigation of heterogeneity. *Br J Psychiatry* 1997;**170**:120–7.
11. Anderson IM, Tomenson BM, Lau J et al. Treatment discontinuation with selective serotonin reuptake inhibitors compared with tricyclic antidepressants: a meta-analysis. *BMJ* 1994;**120**:667–76.

12. Selective serotonin reuptake inhibitors differ from tricyclic antidepressants in adverse events. Evidence-Based Mental Health 1998; 1:50. [Abstract of Trindade E, Menon D. *Selective serotonin reuptake inhibitors (SSRIs) for major depression. Part I. Evaluation of the clinical literature.* Ottawa: Canadian Coordinating Office for Health Technology Assessment, August 1997, Report 3E.]

Second speaker: ALLAN HOUSE

The last few years have seen a staggering increase in antidepressant prescribing in the United Kingdom, which is largely attributable to an increase in prescribing of selective serotonin-reuptake inhibitors in primary care. Prescribing of SSRIs increased five-fold (by volume) between 1992 and 1997 and appears to be still on the up, so that the newer drugs now account for over half of all antidepressant prescriptions.[1]

Although SSRIs account for only just over half the volume of antidepressants prescribed, they currently account for more than 80% of the costs. Suppose a policy of prescribing newer drugs as first line would mean that 70% of prescriptions were for the newer drugs, with 30% of prescriptions (for non-responders) being for older drugs. The additional cost to the National Health Service (NHS) would be £70–80 million at present prices.

As Dr Geddes has outlined, there is no evidence that the newer drugs are more effective than older drugs. Despite flamboyant claims about their lack of side effects, the differences from older drugs in terms of tolerability are small. So what are the grounds for arguing that this striking expansion in their use – with its associated increase in costs – is justified?

The three most commonly used arguments are as follows.

- Randomised controlled trials (RCTs) do not give a realistic picture of the real world effectiveness of newer drugs (although *of course* they give a realistic picture of their greater tolerability). The reason is that in RCTs the older drugs are prescribed in therapeutic doses because the protocol demands it, whereas in the real world they are prescribed in sub-therapeutic doses – either out of ignorance or because of fear of side effects.
- Newer drugs are less toxic in overdosage than older drugs, and their widespread use will therefore reduce the suicide rate.
- Newer drugs have other lower toxicities in therapeutic use, which result in hidden cost savings.

Let's examine each of these claims in turn. First, are newer drugs more likely to be effective because they are more likely to be prescribed in effective doses? Since the dosage at which SSRIs are prescribed is relatively stereotyped, the argument rests on the belief that tricyclic antidepressants are usually prescribed in ineffective doses – that is, in doses the equivalent of less than 125–150 mg amitriptyline per day.[2] Actually, the tricyclic dosages recommended as effective come from guidelines which are based on consensus[3] rather than on a synthesis of the evidence. A recent systematic review and meta-analysis has cast doubt on such recommendations – lower doses of the older drugs aren't as bad as they look in the consensus statements.[4] In the meta-analysis, of patients who were prescribed <100 mg imipramine equivalents 46% showed improvement, of those who were prescribed 102–200 mg imipramine equivalents 53% showed improvement, and of those prescribed >201–250 mg 48% showed improvement. As dosages were increased the rate of side effects increased more impressively than the benefits – from 22% for dosages <100 mg to 30% at 102–200 mg and 37% at 201–250 mg. Surprisingly (to the experts who write consensus statements) when general practitioners prescribe 'low' doses of tricyclic antidepressants they seem to sacrifice little in the way of effectiveness but reduce side effect rates considerably.

Second, does prescribing the newer drugs reduce suicide rates? Here the argument is that a prescription for a tricyclic antidepressant is the equivalent of giving a depressed person the means to kill himself or herself – the so-called 'loaded-gun argument' (a typically dramatic phrase that owes more to salesmanship than to critical appraisal).[5] The best evidence that bears on this question comes from a study conducted by Jick and colleagues.[6] They identified and followed up a cohort of people who had received a new prescription of antidepressants from their general practitioner, with the aim of determining whether the general practitioner's choice of antidepressant was a risk for subsequent suicide. The first important finding was that 94% of suicides in the cohort were committed by means other than the ingestion of prescribed antidepressants. What this indicates is that limiting access to antidepressants that are potentially lethal in overdose will have very little impact on the suicide rate. The second finding was that, after adjustment for known suicide risk factors, the only antidepressant prescription that was associated with an increased risk of subsequent suicide was fluoxetine. In other words, there is no evidence at all from this study to suggest that switching from older to newer drug prescribing will reduce the suicide rate – if anything the reverse.

What about the third suggestion, which is that newer drugs have lower toxicity in therapeutic dosages, leading to 'hidden' cost savings? A typical example is the claim that older antidepressants cause sedation and falls in the elderly. Indeed this does seem to be true; it is a general property of psychotropic drugs (including analgesics) that they are a risk for accidents.[7-9] But recent evidence suggests this is just as true for SSRIs as it is for older antidepressants.[10] The story is the same when we look at road traffic accidents – psychotropics (perhaps especially benzodiazepines) appear to be a risk, but there is no evidence for a difference between newer and older drugs.[11] Of course, all these risks pale into insignificance beside the risk represented by alcohol consumption.[12]

So, if we review the evidence from the best types of study – those that are reasonably well conducted and that make some attempt to adjust for important biases and confounders – we find no grounds for believing that a switch to prescribing newer antidepressants as first-line treatment for depression will lead to better outcome of the depression, will reduce the suicide rate, or will reduce accident rates. Claims to the contrary are based on consensus statements, innuendo, or – that old friend of the partisan – selective quoting from the literature. Given the huge cost differences between the new and old drugs, the former would have to show substantial clinical advantages to justify their widespread first-line use, and they don't.

My own view, however, is that we should go further and favour the older drugs even if the costs were not greatly different. We should always adopt a cautious attitude to new drugs because we know less about their potential disadvantages – both because they may be withheld from us (new drugs are more marketable than old, as long as the image holds up) and because we haven't had time to learn about less common and unpredictable disadvantages. I will give two examples.

- A recent paper has suggested that SSRIs are associated with an increased risk of gastrointestinal bleeding.[13] This may not be a major problem (we can't be sure) but it is inevitable that new problems will emerge with monitoring of longer-term use, and that these will shift the balance of enthusiasm.
- Second, I raise the possibility of dependence as a longer-term problem. It is now generally accepted that some patients develop a withdrawal state when they stop antidepressants; I don't know if it is worse in patients who are taking SSRIs – to me it seems like it but my observations are prone to bias. What I do know is that we shouldn't ignore the possibility that newer antidepressants can generate dependence – rebadge withdrawal as a discontinuance syndrome, reassure ourselves and carry on.

In conclusion, I would like to say two things. First, to remind you that my argument is essentially conservative. To commit the resources necessary to use new antidepressants as first line, we need *convincing* evidence that they are more effective, better tolerated, less toxic in therapeutic dosage, or a realistic means to prevent suicide. There isn't any. The explosion in the use of SSRIs represents a triumph of marketing over evidence-based medicine and as such it is profoundly disappointing.

Finally, a comment on the motion, which implies that the choice for first-line treatment is between older and newer drugs, when it is really between drugs and non-drug treatments. It has been suggested that nearly 3% of the United Kingdom population are taking a prescribed antidepressant[1]; is that desirable? I don't think so, and yet one of the reasons for our continued medicalisation of distress is that we fall for the promotional claim that new antidepressants are harmless wonder-drugs.

References

1. Mason J, Freeman N, Young P. The effect of the distribution of effective healthcare bulletins on prescription of specific serotonin-reuptake inhibitors in primary care *Health Trends* 1998/99;**30**:120–2.
2. Donaghue J, Tylee A. The treatment of depression: prescribing patterns of antidepressants in primary care in the United Kingdom *Br J Psychiatry* 1996;**168**:164–8.
3. Paykel ES, Priest R Recognition and management of depression in general practice: consensus statement *BMJ* 1992;**305**:1198–202.
4. Bollini P, Pampallona S, Tibaldi G *et al*. Effectiveness of antidepressants: meta-analysis of dose-effect relationships in randomised clinical trials. *Br J Psychiatry* 1999;**174**:297–303.
5. Bryan J. GPs unwittingly increase suicide risk. *Gen Practit* 1992;May 22:68–9.
6. Jick S, Dean A, Jick H. Antidepressants and suicide. *BMJ* 1995;**310**:215–8.
7. Ray W, Griffin M, Schaffner W *et al*. J Psychotropic drug use and the risk of hip fracture. *N Engl J Med* 1987;**316**:363–9.
8. Ray W, Griffin M, Malcolm E. Cyclic antidepressants and the risk of hip fracture. *Arch Intern Med* 1991;**151**:754–6.
9. Cummings R, Miller J, Kelsey J *et al*. Medications and multiple falls in elderly people: The St Louis OASIS Study. *Age Ageing* 1991;**20**:455–61.
10. Liu B, Anderson G, Mittman N *et al*. Use of selective serotonin-reuptake inhibitors and risk of hip fractures in elderly people. *Lancet* 1998;**351**:1303–7.
11. Barbone F, McMahon A, Davey P *et al*. Association of road traffic accidents with benzodiazepine use. *Lancet* 1998;**352**:1331–6.
12. Everest J, Tunbridge R, Widdop B. The incidence of drugs in road traffic fatalities. *Transport and road research laboratory research report No. 202*. London: Department of Transport, 1989.
14. De Abajo F, Rodriguez L, Montero D. Association between specific serotonin-reuptake inhibitors and upper gastrointestinal bleeding: population based case-control study. *BMJ* 1999;**319**:1106–9.

Debate chairman's concluding remarks

As I explained at the outset, the idea behind this debate was to present the most up-to-date collated evidence in an unbiased way, for and against the motion, so that you could make up your own minds. It was not our intention to end with a binding vote. However, using my chairman's prerogative, I would be interested in repeating my own little vote. Now to reverse tradition, I want to ask one group in the audience to vote first. You heard me say at the start that the SSRIs get used more effectively than the TCAs, probably because they have been prescribed by female rather than male therapists. But in addition, the evidence that men respond to anything – interpersonal therapy or cognitive therapy, for example – is not there.

So given all of that, I would like to ask the women in the audience to vote first. Should the new generation of drugs be the first-line of treatment for depression?

- **On a simply female vote, those against the motion win.**

Would the whole house now please vote:

- When the whole house votes, the curious thing is that, when we include the men, who apparently do not actually do the prescribing of the SSRIs, **the house votes to prescribe them.**

An interesting outcome!

Closing remarks of the meeting

KIRSTEN STAEHR JOHANSEN

On behalf of the World Health Organization, I would like to thank our collaborators, the International Federation of Health Funds, Harvard Medical School, and the Sir Robert Mond Memorial Trust and all the speakers for their help in making this such an interesting meeting. Over the past few days we have learned may things about depression, not least just how much suffering it can cause patients, their families and colleagues and of the great financial burden it places upon already stretched health services, especially if treated inappropriately and ineffectively. Depression is difficult to prevent but not impossible and we must take heart from the fact that effective treatment is available. We have heard how male depression often goes unrecognised leading in many instances to disastrous consequences. We have also heard of the pivotal role the general practitioner has to play in the diagnosis and treatment of depression. I would also add that in addition to the psychiatrist, the psychologist and other non-medical carers also have a vital role to play. As yet the potential role of payers and politicians in improving the service to people with depression remains unexplored.

It is therefore a challenge for all providers, politicians, payers and the public to ensure that health information systems include indicators for monitoring outcome and cost, in order to allow for comparison, management, accountability and solidarity. I know we can meet that challenge.

Index

Note: Page numbers in **bold** type refer to figures; those in *italic* refer to tables or boxed material